My ♥ Millennium

An Inspiring Journey of a Young Woman Conquering Cancer

*To Diane —
My amazing friend — Enjoy!!
♡ Vicki*

Vicki Bednar

outskirts press

My Millennium
An Inspiring Journey of a Young Woman Conquering Cancer
All Rights Reserved.
Copyright © 2025 Vicki Bednar
v3.0

The opinions expressed in this manuscript are solely the opinions of the author and do not represent the opinions or thoughts of the publisher. The author has represented and warranted full ownership and/or legal right to publish all the materials in this book.

This book may not be reproduced, transmitted, or stored in whole or in part by any means, including graphic, electronic, or mechanical without the express written consent of the publisher except in the case of brief quotations embodied in critical articles and reviews.

Outskirts Press, Inc.
http://www.outskirtspress.com

ISBN: 978-1-9772-7517-2

Cover Photo © 2025 Kate Oelerich Photography. All rights reserved - used with permission.

Outskirts Press and the "OP" logo are trademarks belonging to Outskirts Press, Inc.

PRINTED IN THE UNITED STATES OF AMERICA

*This book is dedicated to my mother,
Barbara, the force of nature I love dearly.*

Table of Contents

Prologue i
Chapter One ~ January 2000: My Millennium Diet 1
Chapter Two ~ February 2000: My Career Challenge 14
Chapter Three ~ March 2000: My Time Off 23
Chapter Four ~ April 2000: My New Career 34
Chapter Five ~ May 2000: My Diagnosis 45
Chapter Six ~ June 2000: My Plan 78
Chapter Seven ~ July 2000: My Move to Mom's 104
Chapter Eight ~ August 2000: My Leave 130
Chapter Nine ~ September 2000: My Wig 153
Chapter Ten ~ October 2000: My Wake and Bake 176
Chapter Eleven ~ November 2000: My Barbados 188
Chapter Twelve ~ December 2000: My Remission! 210
Epilogue 223
Acknowledgments 228

Author's Note

As a newly diagnosed cancer patient at the age of thirty-four, I frantically searched for information on Hodgkin's lymphoma and for survivors to talk to.

As a cancer survivor, I searched for ways to help other newly diagnosed cancer patients and for a means of obtaining closure on my cancer journey.

I began writing *My Millennium* in 2001. Unfortunately, I started researching the publishing process and became sidetracked with life. Over twenty years later, it was not written for my cancer closure anymore, but finishing the book was cathartic for me in other respects, as I relived a very important year of my life. It helped me reflect on my life experiences and my relationship with my mother. Hopefully, my book helps people; and hopefully, you get a chuckle or two.

My Millennium is about my experience in the year 2000. I have included my interpretations of actual situations. A few of the names, dates, and details have been changed for the book. Luckily, I had an extremely detailed journal to help me along the way. I also had medical records and discussions with most of the people in the book to confirm some of my thoughts and remembrances.

Most of the dialog is pretty close to what was said. I have a good memory of the year that was so pivotal in my life. I am sure there are also some things that I chose to forget.

Dream dreams, embrace challenges, pivot, plan, focus, fight, survive, and thrive!

Enjoy!

Prologue

> "If my mind can conceive it, if my heart can believe it, then I can achieve it."
>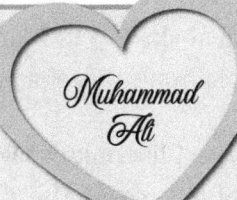
> —Muhammad Ali

My millennium began on December 31 with a serious commitment to change for the new millennium. At thirty-three, I felt like I was at a crossroads in my life and I needed change. I did not fear change; I embraced it. I, being a goal-oriented person, have always made goals for the year, but this was different. I was committed to making a significant change in health, dating, and career.

The first of these millennium changes was to be achieved by what I called "The Millennium Diet." I had gained some weight and was not feeling very healthy. I wasn't huge or anything, but I felt a bit chubby and sluggish. I wanted to lose ten pounds. You could tell I was serious about The Millennium Diet, because I told everyone about it. When everyone knows you are on a diet, it is harder to cheat. That's called accountability. The Millennium Diet plan required me to go on a protein diet by eating mostly protein and limited carbohydrates. I planned to slowly add more carbohydrates into my diet after I lost the desired weight. This way, I could get the weight off quickly with a proven method and maintain my weight once it was lost.

At the same time, I committed myself to running two miles a day, or more, on the treadmill. The plan was to start out fast-walking two miles for the first week, then walk one mile and run one mile, then eventually run two miles a day. The goal of The Millennium Diet was to lose ten pounds and get in shape for my family's annual ski trip in March. Of course, once in shape, I was to magically maintain this shape for the rest of my life.

The Millennium Diet and exercise would help me with my next goal of improving the dating scene. This plan included meeting the man of my dreams as I boogied down the slopes in Colorado looking like the hot babe of the new millennium. Maybe in Colorado, maybe somewhere else, but The Millennium Diet would put me in prime condition to meet the handsome, intelligent, funny, kindhearted man of my dreams. I had a habit of dating attractive, athletic guys who worked at the Board of Trade. There is nothing wrong with that, but I always thought I would meet a nerd like me. Not that I am really a nerd, but I am an electrical engineer climbing the ladder in a big corporation, so I thought I would meet a smart guy from a corporate environment.

I knew I was going to meet this millennium man soon, because a fortune-teller in New Orleans told me I was going to meet this man, get married, and move far, far away—out of the country. The marriage and the move were supposed to happen when I turned thirty-six, so I figured I would meet him soon, and I wanted to look my best when I met my future husband. By the way, I am not overly superstitious, but my overactive imagination liked the idea of meeting this mystery millennium man and moving to a magical foreign land.

Which brings me to my third commitment for change. I had a great twelve-year career at the corporation, moving up the ladder with a promotion every year or two. I had been in the same position for over two years and was ready to move on. The corporation had been very good to me, and I had been very good to it. I was making a decent living, saving money for the future, and belonged to a country club in the suburbs. I was a work-a-holic, which didn't help with meeting my millennium dream man.

There were several career opportunities that were going to open up soon, and I was ready for my next challenge. I was determined to make something happen. The question was, which opportunity was it going to be? My background was in engineering and sales, so I could take my career in many directions with the high-tech corporation. The answer to my millennium career challenge would shake out in the next month or two.

My friend Cate and I spent New Year's Eve together to kick off the millennium. On New Year's Eve, we went to a party at a friend's cottage in Wisconsin with four couples and their kids. We were all spending the night to celebrate and be safe from the crazy millennium.

For months (or years), there had been Y2K talk of systems going down due to computer failure creating dangerous riots in the streets and anarchy—all due to the date change. I heard stories about people stocking up for the winter with food, water, and other supplies. Gun sales had increased tremendously over the past six months. According to some, it was going to be complete chaos. We did not know what to expect, so we decided getting away from it all would be the best plan. On New Year's Day, if we survived it all, Cate and I planned on going back to Chicago to civilization.

Cate and I have been friends since third grade. She is a genuine, athletic, fun redhead who is a blast to be around with her wit and colorful personality. We have been through a lot together over the years, and are two of the last single friends. We played sports together, especially skiing and softball. As two fun-loving, single women, we hung out a lot together. At thirty-three, I tended to still hang out a lot with friends from high school, which was easy to do, since most of them moved downtown to the Lincoln Park area.

I think Cate and I were both wondering what we were doing driving from Chicago to Wisconsin for a New Year's Eve party with all couples and eight little children on the one and only millennium celebration. These were our good friends, and we would have a good time—*and what if the paranoid people are right about the millennium chaos?*

Due to the anticipated nature of the party, we decided to make a few pit stops on the way to Wisconsin from Lincoln Park. We first stopped at my mom's townhouse in a northern suburb, Glenview, for a glass of champagne. My mom was going to a party with some friends. Being a widow going out with all couples, she was in pretty much the same situation as Cate and I that New Year's Eve. As another fun-loving, single woman, my spunky mom was not going to stay home on our one and only millennium celebration night.

Mom toasted the new century in saying, "Happy New Year! May this year bring us all health and happiness!" She was dressed to the nines for her party in a sequined dress.

"And may you find a great dance partner tonight! By the way, you look amazing," I chimed in.

"Yeah, right. Like I'll be doing a lot of dancing tonight," she replied sarcastically.

"Well, you've got a better chance than we do. We'll be hanging out listening to baby stories all night," Cate added glumly.

"Well, you're right. My conversations will probably include a lot more on sports and politics than babies. Although there will be some grandma talk. And you're right. I probably will have a chance to dance with some of the husbands occasionally," Mom said with a smile on her face.

I was sure the sports and politics conversations would be exciting to my mom. She was politically astute and loved sports. She knew more about sports than most men I knew. She read the sports section of the *Chicago Tribune* from front to back every day and listened to sports radio most of the day in the house and car. In fact, she had gotten to know the guys on the radio so well it was almost like they were her close personal friends. They were her buddies.

Mom's love of sports came from falling in love with my dad. When they started dating, she figured she had to learn to love sports because my dad loved sports and had season tickets to Notre Dame football, Northwestern football, the Chicago Bears, and the Chicago Blackhawks. That is when she started reading the sports section every day.

Mom has been a widow since 1994 when my dad died from melanoma at the age of fifty-eight. His cancer had metastasized, and he passed away with fifteen tumors in his brain. It was very devastating to our family and friends who loved him dearly. He had a self-proclaimed nickname of "Bobby Good Guy," which was absolutely true. He was Bobby Good Guy and my hero.

The three of us toasted again, and Cate and I moved on.

We jumped in my Chrysler Sebring convertible and drove to a Wisconsin hick bar on the way to the party. Actually, I believe the bar we stopped at was on the Illinois side of the border, but I would still call it a Wisconsin hick bar. Cate and I decided we wanted another drink before joining the families at the party. Some interesting, unshaven men in flannel shirts with Skoal and Yamaha caps bought us drinks. Unfortunately, these men are not always the ones you want to buy you drinks. As we discussed machines (snowmobiles) and the lack of snow that year, I couldn't help but notice the dip stuck in the Skoal man's teeth. Then I noticed the other man's teeth were rotting away. This was not my picture of my millennium dream man, so we did what a lot of single women would do; we thanked them for the drinks and left.

The New Year's Eve party was at my friend Heather's parents' cottage on Twin Lakes just over the Illinois/Wisconsin border. Heather and I have been lifelong friends, next door neighbors, and roommates. I was always the more studious one, and she was the more athletic one.

Heather and I rekindled our friendship when she moved back to Chicago after academics and golf at Arizona State University. At twenty-four, we lived together in my townhouse and had a fantastic time as young college grads in Lincoln Park. We did a lot of sports together—softball, football, golf, water skiing, snow skiing, etc. Heather eventually married my cousin Kurt, and they had four children. I am the godmother of their oldest child, Jack, which I take great pride in.

Cate and I walked into Heather and Kurt's New Year's Eve party at last. All of the couples had been there a while. You could tell by the buzz. I guess Cate and I didn't really need to make two pit stops. Luckily, the kids were nowhere in sight. Not that I don't like kids. I LOVE kids. They just did not belong at the millennium party. The adults were outside smoking by the bonfire, in what little snow we had. I didn't like smoking but joined the bonfire anyway. Besides, I already smelled like an ashtray from the Wisconsin hick bar.

Dinner was delicious: lobster and filet mignon. Heather and Kurt were the best hosts. We had goofy hats and party favors and enough champagne for twice as many people.

After an amazing two-hour dinner, we played silly games until the ball dropped. The couples hugged and kissed. Cate and I hugged. I went up to bed a little after midnight—the first to go up. *Now that is a first!* A few of the group noticed.

"Vicki, where do you think *you're* going?" Kurt exclaimed as I headed for bed.

"I am bushed," I said wearily.

"You can't go up until you have one more glass of champagne," declared Heather.

"No, thanks."

"But you are usually the last one left standing, not the first one to go down," Kurt said.

"Oh well, things change," I replied as I thought about the change that was to occur during the millennium.

Maybe it had something to do with my commitment to the millennium. No. I was just unusually tired. I crashed on the couch in the game room and contemplated all of the new changes I would have ahead of me this millennium. The year 2000 was going to be a super year for me. I was going to be a healthy, hot-looking woman with the perfect man and the perfect career. I fell asleep with a great big smile on my face.

My millennium was about to begin.

Chapter One
January 2000: My Millennium Diet

> "You are never too old to set another goal or to dream a new dream."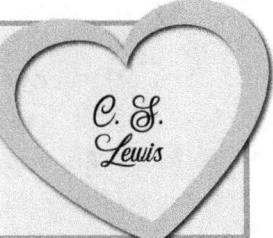
> — C. S. Lewis

January 1, 2000

The Millennium Diet did not start today, because it was a holiday. So the diet started on the second, because the millennium celebration continued for Cate and me. We woke up to chaos in the cottage. It was not the millennium chaos that we had feared but chaos of a different kind. The eight children were running around the house screaming at eight in the morning. Eight at eight was just too much for Cate and me to bear after all the champagne we had to drink. As luck would have it, the families all left early, except Heather and Kurt's family. Heather, Kurt, Cate, and I all lied around on couches and began to watch the college bowl games and drink

Bloody Marys. After a while, Cate and I decided it was time to go and hit the road again. It was time to reenter civilization and find out the level of chaos in Chicago. Everything seemed normal so far.

As we drove back to my mom's house, we talked about the New Year.

"Do you have a New Year's resolution?" I asked Cate.

"Ah, I don't really do that stuff. I stopped making resolutions a long time ago. How about you?" she replied.

"I don't call them resolutions, but I make yearly goals. I have three this year. The first is to work out and lose ten pounds. The second is to focus more on dating and meeting the man of my dreams. The third is to figure out my new career change."

"Vicki, I hate to tell you this, but you always want to lose ten pounds. I think you look great. You should be happy with how you look."

"Thanks, Cate. But I still want to lose ten pounds. Anyway, it keeps me eating healthy. I have been feeling sluggish lately."

I went on to tell her about my career options, and she shared her career updates. Cate worked for her dad's publishing company. She was talking about her potential buyout of her dad. It sounded fascinating. Pretty soon we were back at my mom's house.

New Year's Day bowl games were a yearly event at my mom's house with my mom and me making bets on all of the games. This was a ritual of my dad and me, which was eventually adopted by my mom. Mom was such a sports fanatic that she knew all of the teams intimately and always won when we bet. This year was no different. Back then, most of the bowl games were on New Year's Day, so the games ran well into the night. Cate left my mom and me cheering on teams with all of our hearts when we could care less about the actual game. We wanted to win! Betting a buck a game, we usually ended up with me giving her a dollar at the end. It made for a fun day.

My millennium celebration was over with the Skoal man from the Wisconsin hick bar standing out in my mind as the best catch of the day. Things had to get better than this. *The good news is that it seemed like the millennium chaos seemed minimal. Maybe non-existent?*

January 2-3, 2000

The Millennium Diet began with me walking two miles on the treadmill and going to the grocery store to purchase all the protein I could: chicken breasts, tuna fish, pork chops, steak, four kinds of cheese, eggs, and bacon. On my first day, I had tuna fish, a pork chop, a salad, and eight glasses of water. Day two I had an omelet, bacon, another pork chop, and eight glasses of water. I will not discuss every day's food consumption, but let's just say I was counting my grams, using the treadmill, and keeping true to my word. I was feeling good and ready to go back to work as a new millennium woman.

January 4, 2000

I woke up, ate my egg, walked two miles, and went to work. The first day back at work after the millennium celebration I expected to walk into extreme chaos caused by the Y2K "Millennium Bug" infecting all of our computers and all of our customers' systems. We had a couple of extra days off, just in case there were Y2K issues to deal with on the first through the third. As a sales manager at the corporation, I expected to have many red-flag phone calls from irate customers. I expected systems to be down and lawsuits to be forming. We sold critical systems to public safety entities, utility companies, and other Fortune 500 companies. If their systems failed because of the millennium, lives and money would be lost. We had been upgrading systems for two or three years so that there would be no failures, but you never know with all of the millennium hype. For all I knew, the phone system might fail and the irate phone calls wouldn't get through. That would be a blessing.

The day was the complete opposite of my expectations. It was very quiet. Systems didn't fail internally or externally at the corporation. It was business as usual. There were updates on our sales figures from the end of the year. Everyone was generally pleased, because our division made its sales goals. We were all happy not to come back to chaos, irate customers, and lawsuits. However, we did come back to a management team that seemed to forget about celebrating our 1999 success for very long and was concentrating on sales goals and quotas for 2000 already. That was typical—you were a hero for about five minutes and then it was, "What are you going to do for me this year?" One thing about having a good sales year was that you were assured to have a big quota increase the following year.

As far as my career went, I was in limbo. I had a great twelve-year sales and engineering career at one of the best high-tech companies. I was in systems engineering and engineering management for six years and sales and sales management for six years. It was time for a change. At the time, I managed a North America system sales team with a lot of travel. Actually, it was a pretty good position for me, but I was hungry for more and wanted to move on.

I had been talking to my general manager about several promotion opportunities, but I had my eyes set on one vice president position that I felt like I was perfect for. I had not talked about it with her since Christmas and thought I should bring it up soon, now that it was a new year, a new millennium, and all. Maybe discussing it on the first day back would not be the best idea, so I got on her calendar for the next day to discuss my beloved promotion.

I had a good day at work—no lawsuits, no systems down, no irate customers—and I had a meeting in the morning to discuss my promotion. I went home, ate a steak, and watched prime-time TV.

January 5, 2000

After three days of dieting I had lost two pounds. Two pounds was a start, and I was on the right track. I was determined to keep at it and ate my egg and bacon and walked my two miles before work. This routine made me get up at 5-5:30 a.m., because I had to leave by 7:00 a.m. for my hour commute to work. I had done this commute from the city to the suburbs for twelve years, and it was just starting to get to me. You would think being an engineer, I would calculate the two hours I spent in the car each day and find out how much of my life I was missing out on. I don't think I wanted to know, so I never calculated it. *I never wanted to know that I was missing ten gazillion years of my life just to live in downtown Chicago—the city I loved.*

The meeting with my general manager wasn't very uplifting. We discussed my beloved vice president position. She wanted to fill it within the next week or so and continued to talk about other positions inside and outside the division. I knew that it didn't sound good. She seemed to agree that I would be great for the job, but a little inexperienced. *Inexperienced?* I had twelve years with the corporation without a blemish on my record. I was a terrific manager, mentor, and leader. *If there was ever a position that was made for someone, this position was made for me.* I was driving the strategy for new business opportunities for the division. Whatever I thought about the position, it was becoming obvious to me that my age (experience) would probably stand in the way of me getting the job I felt I deserved.

Besides that meeting, I had a team conference call where I congratulated people on their successes of 1999 and talked about big prospects and changes for 2000. Soon, my first week of the millennium was over and I was glad it was the weekend again. I met Cate for dinner and drinks. Work and its politics were all forgotten by the time we met.

January 10, 2000

Some might say I was successful, but I had still only lost three pounds. I started walking one mile and running one mile today. I was still committed to The Millennium Diet but wanted better results. I was determined.

Today was one of those days you would like to forget. I was in one of the sales vice president's offices talking about business when he interrupted me.

"Vicki, I just wanted you to know that I think you are an extremely talented person and deserve the best here. You are very bright and very valuable to the division. I hope that you stay with us."

I thought this comment was very strange. *Where is he coming from? What does he know? Why is he complimenting me?* There was definitely something going on, and I didn't think I was going to like it.

Cautiously, I replied, "Why thank you. That's nice of you to say."

Suddenly, it was clear to him that I didn't know what he was talking about. He was going to have to tell me himself. "I guess you haven't heard that the vice president position was given to someone else. I am sorry. I thought you knew. I understand that there is another position on the staff that you might be interested in. I think you should take it."

My beloved position was given to someone else. I was going to be given another "staff" position to compensate for my loss. I was bummed. Not only was I upset about not getting my beloved position that I felt I deserved, but also the way I heard about it really sucked. I deserved better than that. I discussed it with my work friends and tried to get a grip. By the end of the day, my general manager called me in her office to tell me. She offered me a lesser position that I felt like I could do in my sleep, but she said I would be very active on "her staff." Looking back, maybe it would have been a good idea to take the job that seemed easier than the job I had, but I wanted the right promotion, the one that I was supposed to have, and the one my skill set matched. *My beloved promotion.* I told her that I would think about it.

The rest of the day was spent preparing for my upcoming sales meetings. I had to get the job out of my head. Next week was a sales managers meeting with my boss in Baltimore. The Leadership Conference with all of the sales managers was in Florida in two weeks. After that, I had my team meeting in Florida. That took care of January into February. In February, there was another sales team meeting in Florida, and there was an Overachievers meeting in San Diego. So there went most of the first quarter. What an efficient way to do business! *No wonder first-quarter sales are always faltering. Oh well, I am going to nice places and going to have a great time.*

January 14, 2000

It was Friday night and my mom's birthday. Since my dad passed away and my sister lived in Orange County, we were left going out on the town just the two of us. We went downtown to Hugo's Frog Bar. While we were waiting for our table, we had a glass of wine in the trendy bar. An impeccably dressed man at the bar leaned over and said, "Hi. What brings you two out on a cold night like tonight?"

My mom and I were both surprised. We looked at him and then we looked at each other. The man was good looking and appeared to be somewhere between my mom's and my age—probably closer to my mom's age. He looked kind of like Michael Douglas. I thought—*what luck on her birthday! Maybe he is interested in her!* I had always wanted my mom to meet someone new. I felt like she was pretty content with me becoming her significant other and always said she already had the love of her life. She was way too young to give up on love.

"We are out celebrating my mom's birthday," I told him, quickly thinking. *Why did I have to say "my mom"?*

"Well, then, you'll have to have a drink with my friend and me. How about some champagne?" he asked with a smile.

My mom jumped in, "Oh, you don't have to do that. Don't be silly. That's not necessary."

The Michael Douglas man looked at my mom. "Do you like champagne?"

"Why, yes."

"Then, Bartender, let's have a bottle of Dom Perignon!"

My mom and I had a glass of champagne with the Michael Douglas man and his friend. We talked mostly about golf. Apparently, the Michael Douglas man went to school and played on the golf team with Jack Nicklaus at Ohio State. The discussion was fun, as we talked about sports. *What a fun birthday for my mom!* I excused myself and went to the restroom.

When I came back from the restroom, the Michael Douglas man leaned over and whispered, "I think you're fantastic, and I was wondering if you would have dinner with me sometime?"

I was a deer in the headlights. I froze. I couldn't speak. *What is going on here? I thought the Michael Douglas man liked my mom. They were flirting with each other. He must be about twenty years older than me. How old is Jack Nicklaus anyway?*

"Vicki, what's wrong?" my mom asked as she noticed the look on my face.

"Oh, nothing," I replied, thinking, *what the heck am I going to say?*

I turned toward the Michael Douglas man. "I really don't know." *Great reply, Vicki.*

"Well, call me when you do know," he said as he put his card in my hand.

My mom didn't know what happened at the time. I did tell her later, though, and she talked me into calling him. I started dating Bill (the Michael Douglas man) on and off. It was not the most romantic relationship in the world, but he became a really good friend. I think our relationship was put in the "friend" category during the first date when I told him that I thought he was too old for me. I am not sure he liked that.

I have not had a real boyfriend in a while. I don't know why. Sometimes I think that my demanding work schedule and travel kept me from meeting men. That is what my mom always said. But I was with men all the time. Sometimes I think I was too assertive, but then I think that I was not assertive or confident enough. Maybe it was my wonderful way with words—like with Bill. Sometimes I think that I was just hard to get to know. *Maybe I should see a shrink in order to help me confirm the New Orleans fortune-teller's prediction of marriage and move at thirty-six.*

No matter what the reason was about I hadn't met that special person, it didn't stop people from saying, "Why aren't you married yet?" or "It's a shame you're not married." I got so tired of hearing about marriage. People acted like I was a failure because I was not married.

The more people asked me about why I wasn't married, the more I started thinking, *Maybe I don't want to get married* or *maybe my career comes first*. The fact of the matter is, I wanted to get married, I wanted to have kids, and I did not want to work if I did not have to. But I had to work, and I worked as hard as I could to afford the lifestyle I wanted. Someday things might be different, but until then, I would work my ass off and succeed at whatever I set out to do.

January 18, 2000

Succeed at everything, except at this diet. I lost five pounds. I was running two miles a day now, but I was still feeling crappy. My joints were sore, and it was hard to run. It had been over two weeks and I had only lost five pounds. *That is stinkin' thinkin'. I have lost five pounds! Yay!*

My friends and I had "dinner club" at a restaurant named Zinfandel. I have dinner club with some friends once a month. There are thirteen of us in the club. We pick a different place every month and eat dinner and gossip. It is a great way to keep up with friends. It's also a fun way to check out the new restaurants. Most of the crew have two or three children, so the single girls lose out on a lot of the conversation. But then again, the married girls live vicariously through us single girls, so it's a wash.

A tall, handsome man with long curly hair approached me at the restaurant bar as I sat next to Heather. He said, "Your eyes are sooo beautiful," in a very French accent. We chatted for a bit, and I found out Christian worked for Arthur Anderson in Paris. Christian and I sat down at our respective tables, and I thought that was the end of that.

Heather, mother of four, kept going on about how gorgeous the French man was. I told her to give it a break. I had forgotten all about him when sexy Christian came over to wish me a happy birthday during dinner. *It's not my birthday,* I thought. Heather had secretly told him we were celebrating my birthday. He wanted to give me a birthday kiss. The next thing I knew, he was giving me a birthday kiss. Not just a birthday kiss, but a real French birthday kiss! *Yikes!*

Soon after dinner, Cate and I went out with Christian and his friends to a blues bar nearby. We went for a night of music and dancing. *Could Christian be the guy from far away?*

He was kissing me in the restaurant before I even knew him. This guy exuded sex. I did not know what to do with him but kept him out in public. At the blues bar, the kissing progressed to my ears. Kind of slobberingly so. I liked him, but not his slobber. It was hard to dance with this going on. *What am I going to do with him? I am not sure about the kissing bandit...*

I thought Christian was good-looking—really quite sexy. But Christian was not my type. I am pretty conservative. I like cute, preppy guys. The girls at dinner club were dying over him—tall, good-looking, athletic body, intelligent, French, and long, blond, curly hair. If only they were on the dance floor with him slobbering in their ears, not knowing what the heck to do with this sex machine who can't keep his hands off of you. Finally, I set the record straight and told him to keep his hands and tongue off. I felt much better once boundaries were set, and he seemed content. Upon departure from the bar, Christian kissed me and said, "A kiss, a kiss, and a kiss again." He then left me that message on my voicemail every week for a month, blowing me kisses from Paris. And that was the end of Christian. *Or is it?*

I know that the New Orleans fortune-teller told me that I would meet a man and move far away—like a different country—but this was ridiculous. I was not moving to France. I did not even like France. The fortune-teller must have been talking about moving to a country other than France. *I wonder which one? I have to stop thinking about this!*

January 22-31, 2000

The kick-off sales meetings began! The next three weeks were filled with sales meetings at nice resorts with golf, presentations, and partying. I decided that I needed to continue my focus on diet and exercise while I went out of town. I didn't want to give up. That meant getting up early, jumping on the treadmill, avoiding all-you-can eat donuts, muffins, cookies and snacks, and limiting alcohol at night. That's pretty hard at sales meetings.

My meetings spanned from California to Florida, because I worked with a lot of different teams. This meant a lot of golf! I played golf in the rain the first day in California. I am a fair-weather golfer, but the guys wanted to play and I didn't want to look like a wimp. Even though my joints ached, I ended up having one of my best rounds ever. *Maybe I shouldn't be a fair-weather golfer?*

Besides fun on the golf course and at night, we actually had real work during the day. We shared strategy for the year and discussed the biggest sales opportunities. Even if you are exhausted, you need to be on your game. It was a good time for me to schmooze with the leaders and work on my career options.

By the end of January, I had gained all of my weight back. Some Millennium Diet! Not only had I gained the weight back, but I was also having a hard time running two miles. I had cut back to walking one mile and running one mile. My knees were sore. This was really rotten. I was going to be out of town again for ten days, and I was at my top weight. *What a swell millennium! I am at my same weight. I have my same job. And I have the same lack of my perfect man.* I gave up on The Millennium Diet and decided to continue trying to run and eat healthy.

Chapter Two

February 2000: My Career Challenge

> "I'd rather regret the risks that didn't work out than the chances I didn't take at all."
>
>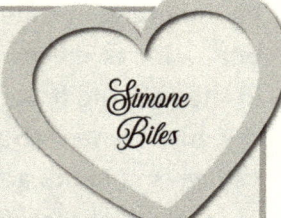
> Simone Biles

February 2, 2000

I had lunch with two vice presidents today. They were discussing two other possible promotions with me, both in project management. One position was Director of System Integration, and one position was a large project management position located in New York. I was promised an apartment in Manhattan. Looking back, these alternatives were not bad. They both used the skills I already possessed and gave me more valuable project management experience. I told them I would think about it.

February 4, 2000

Cate and I went to see Sting at the Chicago Theater. We splurged on fourteenth row tickets to celebrate our birthdays. Our friend, Sue, and her husband, Rohn, also bought tickets. Sue, Cate, and I were so thrilled to see Sting. At dinner before the show, we could not stop talking about how amazing we thought he was. His band, The Police, had been my favorite band in high school, and I was still crazy about Sting. Rohn was probably sick of hearing it and wished he had let the girls go out on their own that night.

The concert was outstanding. Our seats were incredible. Cate and I ran up to the front of the stage to get even closer during the encores. On the last encore, just when I thought I had had the ultimate Sting experience, a girl grabbed me from behind and pulled me up on stage with Sting. I did not know what was happening at the time. I thought Cate was dragging me up on stage. I was in shock. My knees went weak. I looked at him as if I were in love with him and grinned this disgustingly huge grin. He grinned back at me and shook my arm. Not just my hand, but he shook my entire arm. I shook his entire arm. *I am shaking the forearm of Sting! This wonderful, talented forearm muscle is in my hand!* I was still in shock. I could not speak. I wanted to say something profound or intelligent or funny or anything, but I couldn't speak.

I looked out into the crowd to see what it looked like from Sting's point of view with thousands of screaming fans and bright lights. I was looking for Sue and Rohn in the first few rows, but I could not find them. All I saw were lights. I looked back to see where Sting was, and he shook my arm again. Again! I shook Sting's magical, musical forearm twice in one evening. *What a birthday present this is! I wonder if Sting knows it is my birthday celebration. Hey, Sting is from out of the country—maybe we will marry and move to England. I don't think his wife would be too happy about that...*

This whole scene seemed to me to last a lifetime, but it was actually about twenty seconds or less of my life. A bouncer pulled me back down the stairs. It was then that I noticed that my knees were shaking. *Did Sting see my legs shaking? Did anyone else? Did the whole audience see my legs shaking? How embarrassing!* I could hardly walk.

Cate could not believe that it was me on the stage. One minute I was dancing next to her, and the next minute I was the person foolishly grinning at Sting on the stage. She said he was really smiling at me. As we walked out of the theater, I heard Sue screaming through the crowd, "You were on the stage! Vicki, you were on the stage with Sting!" *This birthday celebration is the start of the millennium I was meant to have.*

February 12–18, 2000

I lost two pounds, but I still could not run two miles. I was running one mile and walking one mile. I had officially quit the Millennium Diet, but was still trying.

I went to Orange County, California, to see my sister, Kristen, my brother-in-law, Bryan, and my niece, Kirby, for the weekend before going to an Overachievers meeting in Coronado. I always had such a great time seeing them. They lived on a cul-de-sac with twenty-one children in the neighborhood who always seemed to congregate at their house on the weekends.

The neighborhood knew Aunt Vicki because I came to town two or three times a year for a family fix weekend, usually connected to a work trip. Kristen and Bryan had a wonderful pool with a slide, a tiki bar, and an awesome barbeque pit. They were nonstop entertainers. Kristen and Bryan were really super to me. We actually lived together while I was a senior at Southern Methodist University. Bryan was like a brother to me. They would do anything for me.

Kristen and I have always been very close sisters. Even though she lived so far away from me, we seemed to stay close and had the best time together. Her nickname was Kristen the Kreep, or Kreeps, for short. She has never been very Kreepy, but we all had goofy nicknames, courtesy of my dad. Mommy the Mopes, Kristen the Kreeps, and Vicki the Veeps. I dubbed Dad, Daddy the Dumps. Somehow I hit the jackpot on nicknames! AND, hopefully, I would be a Veep soon!

I had a relaxing birthday weekend by the pool. Kirby's birthday cake really should not have been on my diet, but we were celebrating my birthday and I went running/walking every day. I was officially off the diet anyway, so what the heck.

It was fun to spend time with Kristen and her family. I did not think about my job or about men. I got a call from Bill but had no new male interests. Maybe this fortune-teller was full of it.

I didn't do much schmoozing at the Overachievers meeting, but I did get into another discussion with my general manager. We discussed the four positions I was considering. I had one more interview to do before I was going to make my decision. We weighed the pros and cons of the positions, and I told her I would let her know after the interview. I couldn't wait until this career decision was over with.

When I finally made it home, I had some birthday/Valentine's Day flowers sitting on my doorstep. I opened the card: "To Vicki,

Sending you a kiss from Paris, Christian." The flowers were still alive! I was not crazy about the kissing bandit, but the gesture made me feel special. If only I felt the same about him. *Maybe his slobber isn't so bad?*

February 19, 2000

I was up two pounds from where I was at the beginning of the year. *What's up with that?* I was still having problems running. My knees ached, so I was just fast-walking on the treadmill. It was getting harder and harder to do. This was not at all the way my millennium was supposed to go. *This is supposed to be my year of change, a change in health, men, and career. So far I have zilch.*

My luck changed when I received a phone call from a Canadian friend, Marc. Marc and I mutually respected each other for our achievements and knowledge over the years in business. Marc left his software company to start his own software company to meet the needs of a market that had been untouched. He asked me to join him to run the sales side of the company. I said that I was interested—but I would be expensive.

"Vicki, I have great news for you. The funding has come through, and we are ready to bring you on board as Vice President of Sales for the company."

I was shocked. I couldn't believe this was actually happening. *Will I actually leave the corporation for the start-up? I am so conservative. I don't take risks. Will I actually do it?*

"Oh, Marc, that's wonderful! I am so excited! When can we talk more?"

"I am going to be in Miami next week for a tradeshow. Are you planning on going?" he asked.

"Yes! I will be there! I am presenting. Let's get together," I responded with enthusiasm.

"I will come prepared with an offer. I will send you my business plan for your review. I sure hope it all works out. We could be such a great team."

How exciting! Now, I had a number of positions to think about. I could further my career with the corporation and take a nice promotion, or I start a new exciting career with the start-up that I would own a piece of. At a time when IPOs were making millionaires daily, I could not get the dollar signs off my mind ($$$$$$$). *This is my chance to fulfill a dream!* I always had a dream of owning a company. This was the big change I was looking for in my millennium. I could not wait for the next meeting with Marc, so I started writing down questions, assumptions, and demands.

I called Kristen and Bryan to tell them about my prospective new career. They were so thrilled for me. They asked me about going public and the number of shares I was to receive. I didn't know the details but suggested that the shares I was going to receive could make me a millionaire, if things went well. My niece, Kirby, happened to overhear part of this conversation and grabbed the phone enthusiastically.

"Aunt Vicki, you're going to be on *Who's Wants to Be a Millionaire?*" This happened to be one of her favorite TV shows.

"No, Kirby, I *want* to be a millionaire."

She responded in a very deflated voice, "Oh, I thought you were going to be on the show."

She gave back the phone to an amused parent. It was really interesting how the young mind thinks. I will have to remember not to go to a seven-year-old for career advice.

February 22-23, 2000

I was so excited about my Miami meeting with Marc that I barely prepared for the presentation I was about to give. My presentation was the last one before the group was going to go to a team-building activity, paintball. By this time, no one was listening. I hate presenting to groups that are not engaged, especially when I was not very well prepared myself. With the thought of leaving the company, I was pretty casual in my presentation. I injected humor, but only saw yawns, not laughter. My presentation ended quickly, and the group left for paintball. I left to see Marc.

Marc gave me a verbal offer that I was quite happy with. I negotiated a bit more and asked a lot of questions. Basically, Marc gave me everything I wanted. *But is it worth the risk of leaving my twelve-year career?* I told him that I would commit after I saw the offer in writing, but he gave his verbal and I gave mine. I was basically all in! *Verbally.*

February 24, 2000

I received the offer in writing but did not answer Marc quite yet.

February 25, 2000

I was on my general manager's calendar to tell her which of the four internal positions I wanted to accept. I had been talking to the corresponding managers for about a month now, and it was time to make a decision. She had no idea that I was considering a fifth choice. I felt bad about not being completely honest about the situation, but I wanted to make the decision on my own without external influence. I was thirty-four now, and this was my chance. This was the time to take the risk—no children, no responsibilities. If it didn't work out, I could still go back to the security of the corporation where I had a proven track record, or something different altogether.

I went into my general manager's office with my letter of resignation. I gripped the letter while I started in.

"I have made my decision. What you didn't know is that I was considering a job outside of the company while I was considering the internal positions. I have been offered a great position with a start-up software company. I will be Vice President of Sales for the company. I know I should have told you earlier, but it just happened in the past few weeks when the funding came through. The software product is something I really believe in and think the market has been missing. It is something I can be passionate about. There are fine, quality people from the best software companies in the business recruited for the company. I need to give this a try. It has always been a dream of mine to start a company, and now is my chance. If I don't do it now, I don't know when I will. I have to follow my dream."

Her jaw dropped. She was silently listening to my speech. At the end of my speech, she hugged me. She wished me luck in my venture and told me the door would always be open.

What happened to the begging Vicki to stay? What happened to doubling my salary? What happened to her speech on all of the reasons why I should stay? I was prepared to be strong against all of these things, but I did not need to use my strength. She wished me luck and hugged me. *Doesn't she care if I leave? Was my "following my dream" speech so compelling that she was awestruck and speechless? I guess I will never know.*

That afternoon, I formally accepted Marc's offer and reality hit me. I was leaving. Everyone at work was shocked. *I am climbing the ladder. I am a lifer. Why would I throw that away? Boy, do I have mixed emotions.* People were happy for me, people were jealous of me, and people were sad to see me go. I was happy, excited, and sad all at the same time. I went out with some friends after work to celebrate.

Chapter Three

March 2000: My Time Off

> "Courage is being scared to death... and saddling up anyway." — *John Wayne*

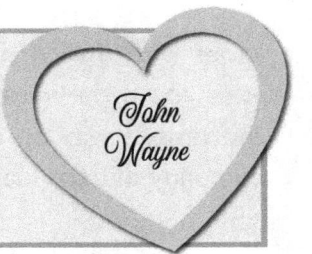

March 1, 2000

Not only did the world survive December 31, but we also survived February 29 without the world going to hell in a hand basket. For some reason, the leap-year date of February 29, 2000, was supposed to be as high risk as the millennium date change. Nothing unusual happened. It was not the end of the world as we knew it.

I woke up today and got on the scale. I was three pounds up from New Year's Day. *What is going on?* I was now walking one mile a day on the treadmill. Our ski trip was coming up quickly now, and I was not the hot babe I was supposed to be. I was not even in shape. Millennium goal #1 was becoming a disaster. Oh well... At least I had my new career to look forward to. Millennium goal #3 was looking good!

Or was it? I questioned myself daily. Today, I was at work and everyone started calling me IPO Vick. It made me nervous. *Am I doing the right thing?* Yes. I had seen the software and truly believed in the solution. I could sell this. There were so many customers who needed this software solution. I had already spoken with several customers in the industry who were very excited about the software solution. *But still, am I doing the right thing?*

I met with the corporation's human resources. I was a little nervous about the meeting because I didn't know what to expect. At the time, I was on a list of "high potential" people of which the company did not want to lose.

"So, Vicki, can you tell me why you have decided to leave the company? You have such an amazing career going. Are you leaving because you did not get the vice president position?"

I reassured the woman that my decision to leave and not getting my beloved promotion were two separate issues. "If I had gotten the promotion, I would not have left, because I would have been committed to the position. If there were no promotion in the picture, I would have left to follow my dream."

I felt that this was not only the politically correct thing to say but also the way I truly felt. She reassured me that the door would always be open and wished me good luck. I think that she was actually excited for me. I think, in a way, they were envious of the enthusiasm I felt for leaving and following a dream. I was kind of happy to hear about all these doors that would be open if things didn't work out, but I didn't plan on needing them.

I had agreed to work until March 13. I had a lot of information transfer to do before then. After that, I was going to Colorado and then take a few weeks off before starting on April 17 with my new company. I had a ton of things to get accomplished between Colorado and April 17. It seemed as though my little break between jobs was not going to be a relaxing break at all. But that was okay. I was making a big change for my millennium.

March 13, 2000

Well, today was the day that I was ending a twelve-year career and moving on to the next. I was upset with my management for not having any kind of send-off for me. I had been to countless retirement parties for people leaving the corporation. *Why can't I have one?* My management told me that they were not happy about me leaving, did not want to celebrate it, and did not want to set an example of celebrating employees departing from the company. I felt they owed me something for the twelve years I worked my ass off. No plaque, no thanks, no nothing after all of these years, just a shake of the hand and a "the door will always be open" declaration. *What a bummer.* Luckily, I had some great work friends who threw me their own party at a place down the street. I soon felt appreciated and forgot all about the lack of appreciation from management.

March 14–22, 2000

My mom and I left for Colorado. I was not the hot millennium babe I was supposed to be. At this point, I had gained five pounds and gave up the treadmill due to my aching knees and ankles. But I was psyched to ski and be free to have a super time at my favorite place. My mom and I had the first day to ourselves, and then Kristen, Bryan, and Kirby were joining us on day two. We stayed across the street from the gondola. We had our routine down and went to our favorite places.

The routine went like this: First, we dropped Kirby off at her lessons. We skied hard during the day from 9:00 a.m. to 3:00 p.m. Then, we picked Kirby up and après skied on our patio overlooking the mountain or at one of the many establishments nearby. Sometimes we hot-tubbed (Kirby and Mom loved this part). Then we went to dinner at one of the many amazing restaurants in town. Finally, we went to listen to jazz or other music, danced, and called it a night.

Once the gang was there, we fell into our routine. Kristen and I were double-diamond skiers, since learning to ski at ages six and four, respectively. We loved extreme skiing and moguls. Even though I was more fatigued than usual, I skied pretty well for being out of shape. The weather was beautiful. We loved sunning in lounge chairs on the top of the mountain with a glass of wine, forgetting about time. Bryan sometimes looked at skiing as an expensive cover charge to God's most beautiful bar. When Kirby's lesson was up, we skied through the trees on all of the kids' trails. She loved skiing with her family.

Mom was very excited about getting home each day after skiing. She could not wait to après ski and hot-tub. For the past few years, there was a teenager in the hot tub with nipple rings and gigantic body tattoos. Each year he seemed to add more tattoos and more rings. He had rings in his nipples, his eyebrow, his ears, his nose, and God knows where else. Half of his body was covered in some kind of tattoo or another. Mom was scared of him, and Kirby giggled at him. Needless to say, we tried not to hot-tub with this fellow, because my conservative family could not control themselves.

Back to millennium goal #2: MEN. I tended to meet men on these ski trips. The ratio of men to women was very good while skiing. Yes, there are a lot of beautiful people, but there are a lot more beautiful men than women. There were also always a lot of foreigners, which made me think my chances of meeting my future dream man in Colorado were pretty high, if the fortune-teller was right. This year I met Steve, from San Francisco. He was a divorced developer who spent a lot of time skiing. California was pretty far away. Some might consider it another country.

Steve and I ended up going to the Sneakers Ball together. This is a fancy annual event, but people are not allowed in unless they are wearing sneakers. Kristen and I worked on finding the fanciest outfit I could find, without breaking the bank. Luckily, I brought my Chicago Bulls sequined sneakers on the trip. I have no idea why. I ended up with nice black pants and a sequined top. Steve and I had a great time at the ball. We spent most of our time people-watching and dancing. The sneakers were really wild at the party.

We were having a really fun time together until we got back to his condo. When we got there, I came down with a severe case of my monthly cramps. I doubled over in pain and was miserable. *What an end to the evening!* We were actually getting along pretty well, and my cramps had to ruin it. I think we were both thinking it was the date from hell. I ended up taking some Advil and falling asleep on his couch. The end of the night really stunk—like a smelly sneaker. I was sure Steve agreed.

I still felt crappy the next morning when I left Steve's condo. As he gave me a kiss goodbye, I knew that the Sneakers Ball was the end of San Francisco Steve.

I should have anticipated the chewing out I was to get from my mom when I got back to our condo. I was in no mood for it. Not only was I thirty-four years old, but also I had not done anything immoral, sleazy, or questionable. If I was going to get chewed out by my mom at thirty-four years old, I would certainly like to have a reason for it. You know some fun, juicy, immoral, sleazy, wrongdoing. But no—I got in trouble for getting my period cramps at the wrong time and not calling. *My lucky millennium.*

"What the hell do you think you are doing staying out all night?! You didn't even bother to call us! You could have been dead in a ditch or something. I had no way of getting in touch with you! You are so inconsiderate!"

"I am sorry. I was sick as a dog with cramps and had a shitty time, okay?"

"No. It isn't okay! What are we supposed to tell Kirby?"

"The truth?"

I jumped in bed and went to sleep. They went skiing without me. Mom didn't talk to me the rest of the day. The following day, she acted like nothing was wrong. The "wrath of Barbara" usually didn't last long, but it was tough. Vicki was out of the doghouse. The wrath of Barbara was over. Life was good once again.

Mom and I went home exhausted but with a nice tan. And, as usual, I felt like I needed a vacation from my vacation. It was a good thing I had a few weeks before I was starting my new career.

March 23, 2000

While I had some time off, my mom gave me a list of to-dos before going to work at my new job. My mom was an extremely organized person. Not only was she good at organizing her own life, but she had taken to organizing my life as well. Yes—I was thirty-four and my mom was giving me to-dos. It was thoroughly annoying. One of the many to-dos before going to work at my new job was to have a physical. My mom convinced me that having my primary physician in Glenview, and not Chicago, was a smart thing to do. If anything ever went wrong, she and the best hospitals were nearby. Looking back, I should have looked at this as a premonition or something.

I went to see her internist. Before he began to examine me, I told him, "I am thirty-four years old and I feel like I am getting old already. I am fatigued and have joint aches in my elbows, hands, ankles, and knees." Then, I told him about my failed Millennium Diet.

He gave me lots of tests and told me, "You are not getting old. There is probably a good explanation for the way you feel. Maybe you have a thyroid problem or something. We will get to the bottom of this." He made me feel good and bad at the same time. *Why should I feel glad that there is probably something wrong with me?*

March 24, 2000

We had my blonde, spunky friend Julie's bachelorette party at my house. Julie was another long-time friend and ex-roommate. I had only met her fiancé once, but he seemed okay. Everyone was happy that Julie was marrying a nice Jewish guy, because Julie had primarily only dated Christians from growing up with us Christians. Jeff was probably the second Jewish guy she had ever dated. Julie and Jeff had already settled down in the suburbs; she was a school social worker, and he was a teacher. Julie seemed happier than ever.

The night of the bachelorette party, Julie and her cousin Dianne spent the night at my townhouse. We decorated my house and had all kinds of rude paraphernalia. We ate dinner, opened presents, and had a limo bus take the party barhopping.

About an hour into the party, Cate and I noticed that we were the only ones drinking alcohol. *Who has dry bachelorette parties?* I guess I do. I had purchased tons of wine, beer, and vodka for the party, and it seemed like no one was drinking it except Cate and me. There were a few pregnant women in the crowd. I was determined to make sure it was fun, booze or no booze.

After barhopping, we came back to my place around midnight feeling exhausted. It seemed like Julie really enjoyed herself. *Maybe we are growing up?* Some of the other bachelorette parties were quite wild. Maybe that was because at those parties we were twenty-something and now we were thirty-something. *By the time I get married, we will probably have a tea party instead of a bachelorette party.*

March 25, 2000

Julie, Dianne, and I went to breakfast. I was not much of a breakfast person, but today was an exception. Of course, I had to do something, because I had no food in my house except leftover bachelorette food. I didn't think that beer, wine, vodka, cake, or hors d'oeuvres would make a good breakfast for my guests, so we went out.

Dianne lived in Florida and was married with twins. She was a riot and spent the whole breakfast telling us about childbirth. Don't ask me now what was so funny, but she had Julie and I howling hysterically until we were crying. I found my partner for the rehearsal dinner. Anyone who can keep me interested in a childbirth story for more than five minutes has me.

The rehearsal dinner was at the Metropolitan Club—a perfect place for a rehearsal dinner on the 67th floor of the Sears Tower. They had a slide show of Julie and Jeff growing up, and all of Jeff's friends made toasts. When it was the girls' turn to toast, we went over our top-ten list of things Jeff should know about Julie before marrying her. Julie loved it. Some of her college friends went into some roasting stories too.

Always the bridesmaid and never the bride—that's me! I spent the evening checking out the inventory of groomsmen. Nothing was grabbing me.

March 26, 2000

Today was Julie's big day. It was also my first Jewish wedding. The rehearsal helped a little bit, but I still did not know what to expect. The bridesmaids were all supposed to meet at the hotel early in the morning to start having our makeup and hair done. I was not too excited about this, since the wedding was not until 5:00 p.m. I had very short auburn hair and did not wear much makeup. There was not much to do, and I didn't want it done by someone else. It typically takes me less than a half hour to get ready. Give me an hour for a special day. I didn't mind hanging around the hotel room, but not for eight hours before a wedding. *How long can you take to get ready for a wedding?* We had already been doing wedding stuff for days. I brought my *People* magazine in case I got bored. To my surprise, the day ended up being really fun as we took pictures of Julie getting ready and reminisced about all of the fun times we had had together. I never opened my *People* magazine.

When it was time to start, Julie and Jeff signed the *ketubah* that meant that they were actually married at that point. The ketubah is a Jewish marriage contract that is signed by the couple before their wedding ceremony. During the ketubah signing, the groom approaches the bride for the veiling. He looks at her and then veils her face. This signifies that his love for her is for her inner beauty. It is a tradition from the Bible where Jacob was tricked into marrying the sister of the woman he loved because the sister was veiled. If the groom does the veiling himself, such trickery can never happen. The actual wedding with the guests was the celebratory part of the ceremony. No trickery here!

The ceremony was beautiful. Julie and her mom had planned it perfectly. Julie looked absolutely terrific and so did her mom. In fact, her mom looked like Barbara Eden. Everyone thought so. The wedding party started calling her Jeannie. That should have made Jeff happy, because Julie will probably look similar to her mom as she ages.

Jeff made a wonderful toast at the wedding. It was funny and meaningful and everyone loved it. I was pretty surprised at how great his toast was. As I said before, I didn't know him very well, but he was really nice. One of the reasons I did not know Jeff very well was because he was quiet. I had never seen him be funny before. Not only was he funny in his toast, but he also seemed comfortable and reached everyone in the audience. *Who knew?*

The two other things that stood out from the wedding were the dancing and the sweet table. The band was exceptional and had us dancing all night until the sweet table opened up. I had always heard about these unbelievable sweet tables at Jewish weddings, but I was unprepared for the table that ran the length of the room. I also underestimated the guests' enthusiasm for the sweet table. I had heard some people talking about how excited they were for the sweet table, but I could not believe my eyes when the crowd on the dance floor rushed the table to get the first dibs on the amazing sweets. This was even after hors d'oeuvres, soup, salad, main course, and cake. You would have thought the group had been starved for three days by the way they rushed the table. By the time I figured out what was going on, the entire wedding was at the sweet table. I squeezed through the herd, grabbed a white chocolate pretzel stick, and ran to get out of the way. Even though I was already full, I wanted to be a part of the traditional Jewish dessert experience.

All in all, it was a great wedding, and Julie and Jeff seemed extremely happy. And I was happy for them.

Chapter Four

April 2000: My New Career

> "Real change, enduring change, happens one step at a time."
>
> — Ruth Bader Ginsburg

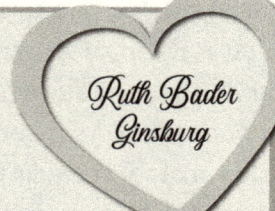

April 1, 2000

I received my physical test results from the doctor today. On the positive side, I did not have a thyroid problem, and my very first HIV test was negative. Not that I was overly concerned about the HIV test, but I had never had one done, and you never know. For all I knew, HIV had caused my fatigue. Whatever the case might have been, I was relieved the test was negative. My doctor seemed to be concerned about my high SED rate and wanted me to see a rheumatologist. Not knowing what a SED rate was, it made sense for me to see a rheumatologist, anyway, because of my joint pain. Maybe I had arthritis or something. So I made an appointment with Dr. Zaacks. Unfortunately, I could not see her for a month. I thought that was a long time to wait, but the alternatives were not any better. My choices were one month, two months, or six months. *I suppose rheumatologists are in demand these days because people are living longer and arthritis seems to be increasing?*

I was still five pounds up from New Year's and not running on the treadmill but running a lot of errands on my mom's to-do list. I wish this was an April fool's joke that God was playing on me, but no, the scale was correct, and I was going downhill in the health department.

Anyway, one of my errands was to see my attorney about a will. I had never had a will or never really thought it was necessary, but my mom thought it was a good time for me to create a will, a trust, and a living will. The living will is one of those oxy morons that basically says you do not want to live if you are a vegetable. I guess it is more of a will to die than a living will. Some of these things I will never understand, but my mom said I should have one, so I set up the meeting with my attorney. As with the physical, I think this was also sort of a premonition or something.

I met with my attorney. We reviewed all of my assets and to whom I would like them to go to if I should pass away. I felt so distant from the situation that I just did all the standard stuff and did not give it much thought. All I knew was that I wouldn't be a vegetable, there was some tax benefit to my benefactors, and I was doing what my mom told me to do. It makes me sick to think of all the things that I do just because my mom tells me to. Yes, I have half a brain and think for myself, but my mom is usually right and I usually just do what she tells me to avoid conflict. *Conflict avoidance—sometimes I think that is my middle name when it comes to my mom.* It was a lot easier than the wrath of Barbara. I have had the wrath of Barbara my whole life, and it is not fun. *I am not sure why I put up with it?*

At night, I went back downtown to meet Cate for dinner. We enjoyed dinner, but we were both tired and went home early. It was a nice night and I walked home. I stopped on my way home at a bar down my street called Marge's to go to the restroom and to see if I knew anyone there. I happened to run into a guy that I met through a friend, Larry. Larry was attractive and outgoing. He bought me a drink and introduced me to his friends. The next thing I knew, Larry and I were dancing to Frank Sinatra on the jukebox and having a fun time. Larry walked me home and gave me a sweet kiss goodnight.

Larry didn't ask me for my number. *What is up with that?* We had a great time, but he did not even ask me for my number or discuss any future plans. I will never understand men. I guess that was the end of that.

April 6, 2000

I received an intriguing phone call today. It was Alan, Larry's friend from Marge's. I was shocked. Larry had not even gotten my number, so why would Alan have it? While we were chatting, I had a flashback of our conversation the other night:

Alan had asked me, "Vicki, what's your last name?"

"My last name is Griesser," I replied.

"That's an unusual name. How do you spell that?" he inquired.

"G-R-I-E-S-S-E-R," I answered without a thought.

I had no idea that he was thinking about looking up my number or that he was even remotely interested in me. That is how much I know about men. I am not perceptive at all. Men are from Mars and Vicki is from Venus, and she doesn't even know where Mars is or that it is a different planet. Vicki is totally clueless about Mars.

Anyway, Alan and I had a long conversation. He seemed really nice. He seemed like just the kind of guy who should be appealing to me. We tried to make a date, but he was going out of town and then I was going to Vancouver. We decided to go out sometime when I got back from Vancouver. My timing was never right.

April 10, 2000

I was making my way through my mom's to-do list. I went through my closets and put together five bags of clothes for the Salvation Army. Five bags of clothes barely made a dent in my closet. I am not very good at throwing away clothes I don't wear. I still have clothes from high school and college. I tried to get rid of as many clothes as possible, but I always think that I am going to wear something again. I have clothes that range from size four through size ten in my closet. I fluctuate so much. I wear all of the sizes. Unfortunately, I was on the higher side these days. In fact, I don't think that I have used size four clothes since my twenties, but you never know.

At night, I stopped by Marge's again and ran into Larry. We were having a lovely conversation, and his charisma was starting to work on me again. I am such a sucker for charisma.

"Alan had told me that he called you."

I was a little surprised to hear that Alan had actually told him. Larry proceeded to tell me all the reasons why I should not go out with Alan. *What is up with that?* They were supposed to be such good friends. I told Larry that it was his tough luck. Alan was the one who called and asked me out.

The next thing I knew, Alan was walking in the bar. *What an embarrassing situation!* Maybe other women had been in this situation before, but I had not. I always wanted to know what it would be like to have two guys fighting over me, but when it was actually happening, I did not like it at all. I wanted to disappear. Some women seem to shine in this situation, but instead, I acted totally uncomfortable—because I was. After a few minutes of uncomfortable chit-chat, I stood up. "Well, guys, I have a big day tomorrow. I better go."

As I started to leave, Alan whispered in my ear, "Do you still want to go out sometime?"

"Sure," I whispered back as I attempted a smile in Larry's direction.

As I walked home, I decided maybe Marge's was not the place for me to hang out. This was more than I could take.

April 13, 2000

Mom came downtown for one of our nights out on the town before celebrating Easter. We went to the Pump Room at the Ambassador East Hotel for dinner. That was one of our favorite places because they had live music for dancing. Not that we danced much, but we liked the food, the music, and the atmosphere. Many times there were famous people who ate there and sat in the Number One

Booth. We kept our eye on the Number One Booth all night, but it was empty.

After dinner, we moved to the cocktail lounge for some cosmopolitans. We were having a nice time listening to the music and talking to an English family next to us when we saw a small unusually dressed woman walk by in a mini-skirt. My mom and I gave each other the look to be quickly followed by my mother whispering, "Who was that? I know that it was somebody like a Spice Girl." I was not quite thinking of a Spice Girl, but I was thinking I recognized her.

"I recognize her also, but I cannot place her." This young woman wore her purple hair in two buns like Princess Leia from *Star Wars*, but more on top of her head. She had on wild makeup and wild clothes. I thought maybe she had just walked off the set of a movie or a spaceship or something.

The unique Spice Girl-looking alien walked by again. I knew I knew her. It was driving me crazy! "Who is that?"

The English woman clued us in. "It is Helena Bonham Carter," she whispered with her beautiful accent.

What had Helena Bonham Carter done to herself? I could not believe it was Helena. We watched her walk to the Number One Booth. Pretty soon there were pictures being taken at the table.

My mom and I talked this over a bit more, and suddenly Laura Dern walked by. There was no mistaking Laura Dern for an alien Spice Girl. She was very tall—looked to me like 6'5" but probably more like 6' tall. Laura was very skinny with a beautiful sequined long dress. She did not belong with Helena, the alien Spice Girl. The group was rounded out with their gentleman friend, Steve Martin. Steve, the comedian in the group, was the only one without a smile on his face. He walked by with his head down and a sharp look on his face. He acted like fans and paparazzi were surrounding their group, when my mom and I were the only ones who noticed them. *What a strange trio they are!*

Mom and I went home to my place after the stargazing experience. We had had our excitement for the night.

April 14, 2000

Easter Day. I loved Easter! Ever since I was a little kid sitting at the top of the stairs with my sister waiting to go on the Easter Egg Hunt, I had loved Easter. It was not just the candy that I loved. It was the hunt. And I loved going to Easter brunch. Even church was better on Easter, because it was such a special time in the Christian religion.

When we woke up, I made my mom go on an Easter Egg Hunt around my house. This was a usual thing to do in our family. We liked to hide things: Easter eggs, Easter presents, birthday presents, etc. I think now the hider has more fun than the hidee, but it was all in good fun.

We went to mass down the street at St. Michael's and then to brunch at O'Brien's. Brunch at the O'Brien's has become a tradition with my mom and me. They have the best buffet, not to mention awesome Bloody Marys.

After brunch, we went to a movie and Mom went home. It was a good day. We pigged out at brunch. Easter brunch, Thanksgiving dinner, and Christmas dinner were the three times when I let myself pig out. There was no such thing as a diet on those days and it felt good. I ate whatever I wanted and forgot all about my failed Millennium Diet.

April 17–22, 2000

I went off to start my new career six pounds up from New Year's Day and totally out of shape. I went to the start-up headquarters in Vancouver to start my new job with a two-day strategy meeting and two days of skiing in Whistler. I loved British Columbia, especially Whistler. I had been there about six times on business, usually with a side ski trip for the weekend. The city is absolutely gorgeous with magnificent views everywhere you look with snow-capped mountains in the background. The sea-to-sky drive up to Whistler is the most beautiful drive I have seen. I had committed to Marc that I would move to Vancouver within the year. Marc wanted all of his top people in the corporate office and I agreed. I looked forward to skiing every weekend.

There were about fifteen people in the start-up now—Marc, five software engineers, six vice presidents, one salesman, and a few administrative people. Okay, so we were a little top heavy, but Marc had recruited a great team so far. He had handpicked some of the best people from the top software companies in the business.

I knew it was going to be an interesting meeting when I got off the elevator and Marc introduced me to one of our investors, Mike. Mike was an extremely handsome man with a nice tan, thick black hair, expensive clothes, and an athletic physique. I shook his hand and felt like I was back on the stage with Sting again. I could not talk, and my legs went weak. I could not say anything intelligent. I just said, "Nice to meet you, Mike." *Why couldn't I think of anything witty or brilliant to say?* Some Vice President of Sales I was. I couldn't even talk. Hopefully, I could speak intelligently in the meeting.

Mike, the babe, ended up sitting across from me in the meeting. It totally took my concentration off of the meeting. I was fidgety and avoided eye contact for fear he could see right through me. Finally, after a few hours, he left and I could concentrate. I was so disappointed in myself for acting like such an adolescent.

The handsome investor was gone, and I was able to be an active participant in the meeting. We discussed product, marketing, and system integration strategies as well as staffing requirements, sales forecasts, and competition. Marc had made a sales forecast that I thought was inflated and much higher than in the business plan, but what did I know—it was my first day. Coming from the corporation's atmosphere with bureaucracy and politics, it was both refreshing and scary to be a part of a start-up that started from scratch. I had so many of the corporation's rules and processes in my head and the start-up had none. There were no standards to go by, so we were making them up as we went along. Like I said, it was both refreshing and scary at the same time. This was going to be a real change for me.

On Friday, we continued the meeting and made our hour-and-a-half journey up to Whistler. We were lucky to catch the breathtaking views before the sun went down. We checked into a decent hotel and hit the bars and nightclubs. Whistler has a great nightlife for all ages: from fast food to gourmet restaurants and from country-western bars to Irish bars to nightclubs and jazz clubs. That was some fun team building for the start-up.

Saturday, all of the non-skiers went back to Vancouver, and the skiers hit the slopes. I was a bit concerned about my knees due to the joint pain and weakness I had been feeling. I couldn't remember the last time that I was actually nervous skiing. I have been skiing expert runs ever since I was a kid. Marc and I had been talking about skiing the expert runs at Whistler, and I doubted whether I was up to the challenge.

As soon as we got off of the gondola, I knew I still had it. I had my strength. I had my style. I had my endurance. I was the expert skier I had always been! It was a great spring skiing day, and I had my stuff. My Rocky Mountain high kicked in and I was happy. Happy, that is, until the end of the day when we had to ski through the heavy slush at the bottom of the mountain. My Rocky Mountain high was over, and my legs could barely get me down the mountain. They were shaking when I took off my skis at the bottom. I guess I was out of shape after all.

We skied again on Sunday. I had my Rocky Mountain highs and lows but was pretty well satisfied with the result of the weekend. I looked forward to working with the quality people that Marc had hired and felt we were on our way with the start-up's strategies.

April 24, 2000

Back in Chicago, a bid request came in from the corporation. They were interested in subcontracting our software on a deal. This could be the start-up's big break. With my connections, we were bound to make this work. We only had three weeks to deliver this bid response, and there was a lot to do. I was already working on a proposal for another customer, so I was immediately busy in my new career. Marc called and he had just received a bid request from another customer on the west coast. They were coming in from all directions. I guess this was a good thing, but I was not quite prepared for it.

I went out with Bill for sushi. It had been awhile since I had seen him. He wore an Armani suit and I wore Gap jeans.

"I am glad you felt the need to dress up for me," he declared as I walked into the restaurant.

"Maybe I don't want to impress you too much," I replied as I kissed him on the cheek. I guess my new life of working out of the house was starting to affect me. St. John designer knits were the outfits of choice on our previous dates. This time, I barely left the house with makeup on. *I can't let myself go like that.*

I enjoyed my nights out with Bill because he made me laugh. The witty banter that occurred between us was not normal for two people who were dating, but then again, our relationship was not normal. I don't think Bill ever got over me telling him he was too old. He was about twenty years older than me. His kids were my age. We always made fun of each other's oddities. He didn't like it because I was just as busy as he was and I was not available when he wanted me to be. It annoyed me that he used to be a golf pro and he wouldn't play golf anymore—not even on a nice day with an average player like me. I belonged to a nice golf club in the area, and he refused to play it. Whatever our relationship was, I liked it. I think we both filled a void in each other's lives and kept each other entertained, but he was not my millennium man.

Chapter Five
May 2000: My Diagnosis

> "If you can't fly then run, if you can't run then walk, if you can't walk then crawl, but whatever you do you have to keep moving forward."
>
> — Martin Luther King Jr.

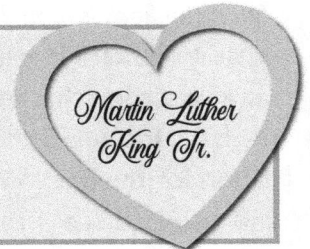

May 9, 2000

I finally met with the rheumatologist, Dr. Zaacks. When I first walked into her office I was a little surprised at Dr. Zaacks's age. She looked younger than me. As I was giving her my five-month history of joint pain, weakness, and fatigue, I kept thinking to myself, *How old is she and how does she already have such a thriving business at the age of twenty-eight or twenty-nine?* For God's sake, it took me a month to get in to see her. I guess I was right. The rheumatology business must have been thriving if a twenty-eight-year-old already had patients waiting over a month to get in to see her.

I was not used to seeing younger doctors. All of my doctors in the past had been older than me. I think, at first, I had a trust issue. *How can she know enough to solve my problem? Am I one of her first patients?* I quickly got over my trust issues when I realized she was very intelligent, **and really** seemed to care. Dr. Zaacks and I got along very well. She tested my hand, ankle, and knee muscle strength and gave me more blood tests. She told me she thought I might have lupus, but she would not know for sure until she received the test results.

What the heck is lupus? I had always heard of lupus, but I did not know what it was or if it was bad. She told me that it was treatable but not curable. I took that to mean that I could be on drugs for the rest of my life. Not fun. Dr. Zaacks gave me some anti-inflammatory medication for the pain. When I got home, I immediately called my mom and sister to see if they knew anything about this unusual disease I might have.

My sister worked for Lexus-Nexus, an online database company for attorneys and accountants. She was a wizard with the internet and looking up information. Quickly, she was feeding us information on lupus, my supposed disease. She emailed me information and faxed information—it just kept on coming. She was like a human library.

I started reading this information that night and soon became depressed. The more I read, the more I figured out that I did not want to have lupus. At first, I was just glad that there was a name to whatever it was that I had and that it could be treated. It was not going to be a mysterious disease anymore. However, the information on the internet had a lot of worst-case examples and didn't concentrate on the best cases. I soon put down the reading and decided I was not going to read anymore until I knew that I really had lupus.

May 12, 2000

I went out to dinner with Cate, to an old reliable Lincoln Park restaurant and bar, Four Farthings. We used to go to Four Farthings for strictly drinking experiences. The bar had older people (thirty-something men) there and was conveniently located. A lot of the other bars in Lincoln Park catered to the just-out-of-college crowd, and Four Farthings seemed to be more like twenty-eight and older. It took us many years of frequenting Four Farthings before we finally realized that they actually had fantastic food as well. Now we go for the food and sometimes for an after-dinner drink or two. Times change.

And sometimes times do not change. Cate was on tempo with her great sense of humor and was directing it toward our waiter, whom she had a slight crush on. Okay, so maybe the waiter was about ten years younger than us, but she was having fun and was really on a roll.

In between flirtatious visits with the waiter, I tried to tell Cate what was going on with me health-wise. I had not told any of my friends about my problems and felt kind of stupid telling them. I didn't even know that there was anything really wrong with me, but my joint aches were particularly bad that evening.

"See, Cate, I can't even make a fist." I showed her that my hand was not strong enough to make a fist. That was the first day that I realized that I couldn't make a fist and squeeze a finger with my hand. "I can't squeeze your finger," I said as I tried to squeeze her finger.

I knew I had problems turning off lamps, but I did not realize I could not even squeeze a finger. Dr. Zaacks had me squeeze her finger a few days ago and I could do it. I know it sounds silly to go on about squeezing a finger, but try it. It is a simple thing to do and I couldn't do it. I couldn't close my fist.

"Awe, Vick. That's not good. What does the doctor say?"

"It could be lupus. She's not sure. I am waiting for test results to come back."

"Let me know if there is anything I can do to help. Keep your chin up. Hopefully, it's nothing."

"Let's hope," I replied with a forced smile.

May 14, 2000

Today was Mother's Day, and my mother was in California with my sister's family. Cate graciously invited me to go out with their family for Mother's Day. I had intended on joining them, but I was bushed. I felt like such a complainer, but my joints ached and I was exhausted. Besides, I had three proposals to work on for the start-up. I decided to work instead. Fun.

At night, my knees and hands felt like they were on fire. I had to remember to tell Dr. Zaacks about this. *Is this lupus?*

May 15, 2000

I woke up at 6:00 a.m. and started work on my proposals. I had so much to do in such little time. My hands were aching again, especially the more I typed. I called Dr. Zaacks to give her an update. *What a caring doctor!* She always called right back. I have always felt genuine concern from her. She gave me a prescription for Prednisone, which she thought would help me. She did not have the test results back yet to tell me if I had lupus or not. I walked down the street to Walgreens and prayed the new medication would help. The rest of the day and night I worked on my proposals, emails, and conference calls.

May 17, 2000

Dr. Zaacks received the test results. I did not have lupus. *What a relief!* My SED rate was still skyrocketing, but I did not have lupus. She made an appointment for me to see a neurologist the next day. She was keeping things moving along and I was glad, because I was getting notably worse every day. I was still working on my proposals but having a hard time on the keyboard. I also noticed that I was having a hard time getting up and down the stairs. I was pulling myself up the stairs with the railing. On the way down, I had to grip the railing tightly so that I would not fall. Even when this was happening, I was in total denial that something was *really* wrong with me. I still thought I had arthritis or something and would get some medication and feel better.

My denial lasted until the night came. Then paranoia set in. At night, my hands and legs would throb and burn. I started to wonder what I would do if I woke up in the morning and couldn't walk. *What if I become paralyzed? What if I cannot get out of bed? Who will I call?* My mom was out of town. After much deliberating, I decided that I would call Heather. Although she lived in the suburbs, she didn't work and could throw the kids in the car and come downtown. I had it all planned out. I put the phone close to me in case I needed to call her. Then I spent the next fifteen minutes trying to decide whether or not to call her that night and tell her that she was my emergency choice. I looked at the clock and figured she had been asleep for two hours by now and thought that might be a bad idea, especially since she had three kids under the age of four.

May 18, 2000

I was not paralyzed! I got out of bed and on the scale this morning. Not good news. I was up eight pounds over my weight on New Year's Day. I was so frustrated. I wrote down everything I had eaten that week and could not understand it. I gave up. It was not worth the worry. So, once again, The Millennium Diet was a failure. I know I officially quit the diet months ago, but I kept going back to it. I gained eight pounds instead of losing ten, and I could barely walk instead of running two miles a day. Oh well, at least I had my new career that was going to make me rich.

Without much explaining, I dropped my proposals in my boss's lap and went to a neurologist appointment with Dr. Randall. I think something in my head told me immediate knowledge transfer was called for on my proposal work, because I was going to be tied up for a while.

Dr. Randall walked in the office, and he looked even younger than Dr. Zaacks. I really felt old. Physically and mentally. He had just as good of a bedside manner as Dr. Zaacks and he was quite cute. He examined me thoroughly and I examined his ring finger. *Damn— married*. Oh well, he was probably too young anyway.

During his examination I noticed I could not walk in a straight line or on my toes or on my heels, besides the rest of my problems. In fact, I could barely move my ankles at all. Dr. Zaacks came in during the examination, and they were both baffled. They decided that I should have another blood test today and an EMG test tomorrow. I had never heard of an EMG. I had heard of an EKG, but not an EMG. Dr. Randall explained that it was an electromyography (EMG), a muscle and nerve conduction test. He said that some people thought it was no big deal and other people thought it was like sticking your hand in a toaster. I was hoping to be one of the no big deal kind of people.

After the appointment, I went to my mom's house to spend the night. She had just gotten home from California and was very upset that she was not around during my downfall that week. I reassured her that everything was going to be all right, but my paranoia came back again that night. At least this time I was at my mom's house and could just yell out if I became paralyzed and could not get out of bed. *This fear of being paralyzed has to go!*

May 19, 2000

I woke up, and again I was not paralyzed, but I could not move my feet at all. My toes and ankles were dead. I guess I was semi-paralyzed. I was numb up to my thighs now. I was glad to be seeing Dr. Randall again today, because I was much worse and walked like a duck. That is the only way to explain it. Since I couldn't move my ankles, I had to point my feet outward to have balance to walk and I walked like a duck. My mom freaked.

After breakfast, Dr. Zaacks called. "Vicki, I want to admit you into the hospital."

My heart started pounding. I guess this was serious. My denial was still kicking in even with my duck walk, but reality finally hit when she wanted to admit me.

She said, "Your blood test came back with multiple irregularities. Your red blood cells, white blood cells, and SED rate are off, as well as having blood in your urine. I want you to be admitted and have an EMG and an MRA done today before the weekend comes. Also, I might start treating you with high doses of steroids before your condition gets worse."

I explained the situation to my mom. Again, Mom freaked.

We packed a bag and went to the hospital. I felt both relieved that finally we would figure this thing out and scared that I would be stuck in the hospital all weekend without much action. Dr. Zaacks said that we would get as many tests done that day as possible.

My mom happened to volunteer at the information desk at the hospital on Thursdays. She called it her "job." She knew just where to go and what to do. I waddled up to the desk to register.

At the registration desk, the woman shoved a bunch of papers at me to sign. "Please read and sign these registration papers. Do you have a living will?"

Now, it was my turn to freak out. My heart pounded and I thought, *this is it. I am going to die, and they know it.* I panicked. "Uh, I have a living will at home, but it isn't signed. Should I drive back downtown and get it? Do I need it to register?"

The woman replied, "Don't worry about it. Just indicate your wishes on the form. Do you want to be visited by a priest or minister?"

Again, I panicked. My father had last rights read by a priest in the hospital, and I took this to mean that I might need last rights. I didn't think I was dying. Maybe this registration person knew more than she was letting on. Maybe Dr. Zaacks knew what I had and therefore the registration person knew my diagnosis before me. I was holding on to the registration desk trying not to fall. I was not worried about being paralyzed anymore. I was worried about dying.

"I don't think so," I said in a feeble voice.

Now thinking back, I should talk to those registration people about their procedures. This was entirely unacceptable to make a perfectly healthy duck-walking individual switch their paranoia from paralysis to death with two questions. My mom and I went up to my room.

I was assigned a room with a woman who looked like she was 120 years old. She had all kinds of tubes in her and was breathing very slowly and loudly. My mom rushed back to the nurses' station to request a private room. They said they would work on it.

A nurse came in to check my vital signs and give me my hospital gown. My mom tried to explain to her that we wanted another room and the nurse babbled something back. Neither of us understood. She just kept checking my vital signs.

I tried this time. "Are there any other rooms available?"

She replied, but all I heard was, *Mumble, mumble, mumble.*

We shrugged. The nurse kept talking, and we did not understand a word she said. This whole experience had me so nervous and on edge. I was scared. Then the nurse started pointing at the hospital gown. She pulled my mom out of the room, and I guessed that I was supposed to put on the gown. I undressed down to my underwear, grabbed the gown, and could not figure it out for the life of me. There I sat, a half-naked engineer, and I could not figure out how to put on a hospital gown. I wasn't a dumb person. I thought I must have been dying, because this was too weird. I had lost it. I couldn't figure out how to put on a hospital gown.

Finally, Dr. Zaacks came to the rescue. She walked in to find me half naked, fumbling with the gown. She took it and could not figure out the buttons either. Okay, maybe I was not losing it, but I was still half naked and gownless. I sat there half naked for several minutes listening to the old lady breathe. Soon Dr. Zaacks found me a new gown. She found me a gown that did not require any thinking or experimenting. Dr. Zaacks told me that Dr. Randall would be by soon to give me the EMG, and I would have a magnetic resonance angiography (MRA) later. I would probably start with high doses of steroids that evening.

Luckily, after I had the gown on, cute preppy Dr. Randall walked in with his nurse. He rolled in this big machine with a computer. He described the test to me and began to zap me. This was not so bad. He shocked me up and down my legs, feet, arms, and hands. It was uncomfortable, but it was not like sticking your hand in a toaster. Of course, I had never stuck my hand in a toaster to know what that would feel like, but this was not bad.

My neighbor started to wake up during the test. She was really moaning, so Dr. Randall went to see what was up.

"Get these tubes out of my nose!" she cried out.

"You need those tubes to breathe. You need to breathe," Dr. Randall replied.

"Get these tubes out of my nose. I don't like them!" she screamed again.

"You need them to breathe. You *do* want to breathe, don't you?" he asked in a calm voice.

"No! I don't!" she responded.

"Well, you need to breathe to live. You want to live, don't you?"

"I guess so." And she went back to sleeping loudly.

I thought this was my big chance. I asked Dr. Randall if he could help get me another room. *What if she does this all the time? What if that loud breathing keeps me up at night? Or what if the loud breathing stops in the middle of the night? What if she dies in the middle of the night? What am I supposed to do?* He told me that he would work on it.

Suddenly, we continued my test without my knowledge. Unbeknownst to me, we had finished the nerve conduction test and were proceeding with the muscle test. The test started with one large poke in the thigh muscle with a needle. "Ouch!"

I did not expect that. After he poked me, he kept the needle in and asked me to flex my muscles. The more I flexed my muscle, the more it hurt. I don't mind needles for drawing blood or shots, but needles in your muscles are a different story. That really hurt. My mom was not doing well with it either. She could see the pain on my face as I screamed. I was in such pain, I didn't even notice if my screams woke up my neighbor. After he was finished puncturing my thigh, Dr. Randall moved to the shin and punctured my shin muscle. By this time, I was getting light-headed, and sweat was dripping off my nose and down my back.

"How many more times are you going to puncture me?" I screeched.

"I have eight more locations," he said.

I fell back on the bed and almost passed out. I did not think that I could make it. This was much worse than a toaster. I kept thinking to myself, *Give me the toaster! Give me the toaster!* The next eight locations went faster, but the last location was the worst one. It was my thumb muscle. I screamed one last time.

I was so relieved that it was over. Dr. Randall told me the test was normal. All of that pain and nothing new. I was normal. *I guess I should be relieved?*

Next, a gurney was wheeled in to take me to the MRA test. The MRA is an MRI test that looks at your arteries. Now the doctors were thinking that I might have a disease called vasculitis. From my information from the human library in California, vasculitis was similar to lupus, except worse. Another incurable, but treatable disease. Again, I didn't want to know too much until I knew I really had it.

This was my first time being in an MRI machine. I was having the chest, abdomen, and pelvis examined, so it took a long time. I think I was in the narrow, closed-off machine for an hour and twenty minutes. Luckily, my mom had given me some tips. She told me to keep my eyes closed and imagine myself playing golf at the country club. I knew the course well enough to go through the eighteen holes in my mind, so I thought this would work.

As I slipped into the machine I closed my eyes and imagined myself walking up to the first tee. Of course, I had a nice drive. Then, I started walking down the fairway. I was about to take another swing when suddenly the MRI machine started making these machine-gun noises in my ear. *How am I supposed to concentrate on my golf game with all of this noise in my ear?* Suddenly, instead of the nice, peaceful golf game, I was in a war fighting the enemies with a machine gun. Don't ask me what war or with whom we were fighting, but I was kicking butt. When the noise went away I went back to my golf game. That is how it went for most of the test. I ended up having a good game. The noise threw me off a bit, but I shot a 101. Then, I went on to go skiing. I skied down slope after slope. When the test was over, I had played a round of golf and skied most of the mountain. Not bad.

After I got out of the machine, my mom asked me, "What were you thinking about during the MRI?"

I told her, "I took your advice and played a round of golf and skied."

"What did you shoot?"

"101."

She snickered. "I cannot believe that in an imaginary golf game, you didn't play better. You should have broken 100 or gotten a hole-in-one when you had the chance!"

I guess she had a point, but I was hitting the ball in my imaginary golf game the same way that I always hit the ball with the exception of the noise interruptions. She was right. I decided that next time I would make myself play better. I was going to kick some ass.

When we arrived back on my floor, we had the good news that I had been moved to a private room. Actually, it was a semi-private room that did not have any roommates in it yet. I was relieved not to have to sleep with the older woman. I had a long day.

My dinner was waiting for me in my new room. Mom and I shared my dinner. This was something that became a habit. The hospital serves you enough food for two, so we split all of my meals. The hospital food was actually pretty good. I had always heard that hospital food was so awful, and that was not my experience at all.

After dinner, my mom went home, and the nurse gave me 1000 mg of steroids in my IV. Even though I was exhausted from the day, the steroids kept me up most of the night. I was wired but feeling good. I started watching Nick at Nite on Nickelodeon. It reminded me of when Kristen, Bryan, and I lived together my senior year of college. Since Kristen was working, the college kids, Bryan and I, watched Nick at Nite after coming home from parties or bars, while my sister was asleep. We usually fell asleep with the TV on and eventually made it to bed. In the hospital, I watched *Gilligan's Island*, *Happy Days*, and *All in the Family*. The next day I was so excited to tell my mom about all of the episodes. She wasn't interested.

May 20, 2000

Promptly, at 6:00 a.m., a nurse came in to draw blood. I found out later that I was to receive this 6:00 a.m. stabbing every day. Nice wake-up. The sun was barely up and breakfast was not until 8:00 a.m. *What am I going to do for two hours?* I looked outside to see the birds chirping and the buds blossoming on a tree nearby. I had a room with a view. I tried to go back to sleep. Then, another nurse stopped by at about 6:45 to check out my vital signs. At 7:30, a doctor stopped by to examine me. At 8:00, they came to change my bed. At 8:15, breakfast came. I felt like a whole day had passed by the time it was 9:00 a.m.

Good news! I could move my feet. Not a lot, but it was a huge improvement. Those steroids probably kept me from becoming paralyzed. Really. I waddled into my bathroom to clean up before my mom came by. Yes, I was still waddling.

Around 9:30 a.m., I started receiving phone calls from friends. My sister had called a few of my friends to tell them I was in the hospital and couldn't walk. A few of them were shocked to hear the news, because I hadn't told anyone about my health problems except Cate. They all made plans to visit me.

I was still wired from the steroids, so having my friends visit was like having a party in the hospital. They all brought me gifts and flowers. Heather and Kurt, Cate, Julie, and Sue all came to visit the first day. They took turns rubbing my feet, because they were freezing from a lack of circulation. Even with two blankets wrapped around them, they were still freezing. We laughed, told stories, and talked about how sad it was that it took someone getting sick to bring us together like that. We shouldn't take things for granted.

Nothing much else happened that day, or the next. I had another 1000 mg of steroids in my IV, which kept me up watching Nick at Nite again.

May 21, 2000

I had the 6:00 a.m. wake-up again. I had an established routine now. My mom always came after breakfast, around 9:30. She would tell me about the people who had called asking about me. My phone was ringing a lot as well. My room looked like a florist shop by now. I had beautiful arrangements that were sent from my friends, my mom's friends, and family. The volunteers just kept bringing them in. The thoughtfulness from friends and family really made me feel good. It feels so good to know that people care.

More friends came to visit, and I still had my steroid high. In fact, they gave me another 1000-mg IV. My mom ran off to see a play with a friend of hers, and I was hanging out with friends watching TV. This was not so bad. I was just worried that they would give me a roommate sometime. I told the nurse it wouldn't be a very good idea to put someone in with me, because of all of the constant flower deliveries, visits from friends, and TV watching. The nurse agreed but could not guarantee anything.

As luck would have it, the paramedics brought a woman with a terrible migraine into my room at around 4:00 p.m. Panic spread over me. The nurse saw the panicked look on my face and ran to get the head nurse for our floor. The head nurse was steaming as she entered the room.

"Whoever told you this was a private room?" she barked at me.

"No one." I shrugged.

"Well then, why do you think you can tell these people they can't bring this woman in here?" she bellowed.

"I never said they couldn't bring her in here. But I don't think that it would be a very good idea to put a woman with a migraine in the loudest room on the floor, if you can avoid it," I responded.

The nurse sneered at my visitors and took the patient out of *my* room. Later, the nice nurse came back and said they were moving me into a private room that they reserved for patients who can't be contaminated. She said it could be temporary, but I would have a better chance of keeping my privacy, if I was moved.

After I was moved, I had my privacy so much that I think they forgot about me. They stopped coming in to check my vital signs. They stopped coming in to change the water or the sheets or clean the bathroom or take out the garbage. They even forgot to give me dinner. Finally, at 8:30 p.m. I buzzed the nurse and told her they had forgotten to feed me. She apologized and scrambled around to try to find something to give me to eat at that late hour. I was happy to have my own room but quite sad to feel neglected. I guess I missed all of the attention I was getting earlier.

I ate a sandwich and watched TV. Nick at Nite kept me entertained, once again.

May 22, 2000

It was business as usual in the morning: 6:00 a.m. stabbing, 6:45 nurse visit, 7:00 doctor visit, 7:30 sheet changing, 8:00 breakfast. Today was Monday and a big day for me. The doctor informed me that I was scheduled for an echocardiogram to check my heart, because it looked enlarged on the x-ray. I was also scheduled for a muscle and nerve biopsy to check for vasculitis. Since the weekend was over, the hospital was hopping. I was finally getting some action. My mom came just before they took me for the echocardiogram. She had a lot of sitting around to do that day.

The echocardiogram was no big deal. The nurse rolled this device over my chest, and she could see my heart beating. It was normal.

I was a little more nervous when I went down for the muscle and nerve biopsies. The doctor was going to make an incision at the bottom of my right calf muscle and slice off a piece of my muscle and my nerve. The doctor happened to be a member from my country club who I didn't know very well. I didn't want to act like a wimp. I tried to be as brave as possible for him. If I didn't know the doctor, I would have shown my true terrified colors.

I lay on my stomach on the operating table and was wishing for medication. Any kind of drugs would have helped.

I asked the nurse, "Can I, please, have some medication?"

She replied, "I'm sorry. The doctor wants you to be alert for the procedure."

I was gripping the table with all my limited strength. The nurse put on Van Morrison and we were ready to go. The doctor gave me a local anesthetic to numb the area. I did not feel the first incision much. The muscle biopsy was no big deal. Then, the doctor tried to find the correct nerve to biopsy. He kept touching two different nerves in my leg, and my leg would shoot out each time he touched a nerve.

"I'm sorry. I don't mean to kick you!" I yelled.

It felt like the nerves were being put in a light socket. Each time my leg shot out I apologized for kicking the doctor. I really wasn't sorry though. I was scared that I would kick him, forcing him to slice off my ankle by accident. Then, he would be the one apologizing. I kept listening to Van Morrison, picturing my ankle being sliced off. It was not a pretty picture.

The doctor finally chose the correct nerve, sliced a chunk of it, and my leg kicked out one final time. Not being able to see or feel my calf, I asked him, "Am I okay?"

He told me, "I got a clean slice and everything should be fine. It will be sore and numb for a few weeks. There is a good chance that your ankle and foot will be numb permanently." *Super.*

I was wheeled back to my room and hung out with my mom the rest of the day. Dr. Zaacks and Dr. Randall stopped by to see how I was doing. Besides my newly sliced leg, I had improved a great deal over the weekend. The high-dose steroids seemed to have helped a lot. They scheduled an occupational therapist to come see me the next day. Hopefully, I would get the biopsy results the next day as well.

May 23, 2000

The nurse had to change my sheets twice overnight, because I was having night sweats. I also had to change my gown. It was soaking wet. *When did these night sweats start?* I had not noticed them before. My hair was sopping wet. *How strange.*

I told my doctor about the sweats when he came to see me. He said he would let me know as soon as they had any biopsy results back.

My mom went and played golf in the morning. I had the morning to myself and my staff of nurses and doctors. I was coming down off of my 1000-mg-a-day steroid high and was very emotional. I just wanted to figure out what this illness was. Anything would make me sad. I watched TV and cried at things that were not even sad, like sitcoms.

The occupational therapist came by to visit me. She mostly dealt with hands. She gave me exercises to do with my hands. As I tried to do the exercises, I started crying uncontrollably. I was so emotional. I couldn't do the exercises and couldn't stop crying. I felt like such a fool, because I couldn't do the exercises and couldn't stop crying. Then, I couldn't stop laughing at myself. I laughed and laughed until I was crying again. I am sure I looked like an insane person to the occupational therapist. She probably left my room recommending a different kind of therapist for me. Something more along the lines of a psychotherapist.

My mom came to the hospital around 2:00 p.m., and we watched a movie on the Turner Classic Movies channel. This had become a habit of ours. I can't tell you how many TCM movies we saw in the past week. I was becoming an authority on classic movies.

Dr. Zaacks came by around 5:00 p.m. to tell me they had gotten the biopsy results back and I did not have vasculitis. I was a bit surprised since vasculitis is the swelling of arteries and lymph nodes; it made sense to me. I felt like my circulation was bad. Since I was still coming off of my steroid high, I started crying at this news. I didn't even know if this was good news or bad news, but the no news was upsetting. I just kept crying. I felt like I was back at square one.

We decided I would have a CT scan the next day to see if anything popped up there. I was resigned to the fact that we might never figure this thing out. I had a depressing evening but slept better. I didn't even need Nick at Nite. However, I did need my sheets changed twice again from the night sweats.

May 24, 2000

It was business as usual in the morning. I discussed my disappointment with the doctor during his 7:00 a.m. visit. He lifted my spirits by telling me that I really didn't want to have vasculitis. It is a terrible disease that cannot be cured. He felt confident that we would figure out what was wrong with me. I felt much better after talking with him.

Luckily, I still had my private room. Friends and family kept coming, and my room still looked like a flower shop. My mom even took some of the flowers home, but the room was still jam packed with flowers. Cate and my friend Robin came by at lunch today and we had a nice visit. They gave me books and magazines. I couldn't concentrate or focus enough to read a book, but magazines I could handle. You don't need to focus much on magazines. Magazines are a great hospital gift.

Then, Heather came by with her kids. Heather had come by almost every day. The kids were not allowed in the room, but she snuck them in anyway. Jack, Hannah, and Chloe were absolutely fascinated with all of the machines and buttons in the room. They were not allowed to touch anything except the bed controls. Soon they were all on my bed making it go up and down in all sorts of directions. We were having so much fun riding the bed, I was sure the nurses could hear the fun all the way down the hall. Heather gathered her kids and left as I was being wheeled down for my 3:00 p.m. CT scan.

I had a chest, abdomen, and pelvis CT scan with an injection. I am not sure what they inject you with, but I guess it helps them read the scan. CT scans are simple compared to MRIs, except the injection makes you feel like you are going to go to pee on the table. This scan was about fifteen minutes long compared to the hour-and-twenty-minute MRI. The nurse told me that I would have the results the next day.

I went back to my room and started watching TCM with my mom when Dr. Zaacks walked in. She gave me the same old tests to check out my hands and feet and asked how I felt. It was all very routine, until she told me that they had the results from my CT scan. I wondered how they had the results already since I was told they wouldn't have them until tomorrow. I had just come back up from having the test.

She held my hand, looked me right in the eye, and said, "They found two tumors in your chest: one large tumor surrounding your heart and another one higher up in the middle of your chest. It is probably a lymphoma of some sort—either Hodgkin's lymphoma, non-Hodgkin's lymphoma, or thymoma. We would like to take a biopsy to see which kind of cancer it is."

My mom and I were in shock. She sat down on the bed with me. The doctor was still holding my hand and wiped a tear from her eye. *What a difficult thing to have to tell someone.* I didn't know how to reply. We were stunned. I didn't know what to say or how to feel. I had this big feeling of numbness sweep over me. Usually I have my wits about me and ask all the right questions, but I was dumbfounded. I think my mom was dumbfounded as well.

Finally, I asked, "Are they sure?"

"Yes."

"When should I have the biopsy?"

"We are trying to schedule it for tomorrow. The thoracic surgeon should come by in the next hour, or so, to meet with you. He is the best. He is a wonderful surgeon. You will really like him. I just wanted to make sure we spoke before he came by."

We talked a bit more, and she left the room. I guess someone reads the CT scans immediately, and if something stands out, they immediately call the doctor. I guess, based on schedules and/or bedside manner, they decided Dr. Zaacks was the best person to tell me. Either that, or they drew straws, and she lost. Anyway, I thought Dr. Zaacks was a very caring doctor and handled it very well.

For some reason, as soon as the doctor left the room, the phone rang off the hook. Everyone started calling. It was like they knew what had just happened. We didn't answer the phone. We didn't want to talk to anyone yet. I think we were still in shock.

I have cancer. This was the millennium from hell. I think I had always known that I was going to get some form of cancer—someday. My dad's family had a lot of cancer in it, but I was only thirty-four. I thought I would get cancer later in life. *This is not supposed to happen now. I have so many other responsibilities. I have my new career.* I knew nothing about lymphoma or how bad it was. I knew it was not good to have cancer spread to your lymph nodes, but what was lymphoma? We would have to get the human library started on this one.

My thoughts turned toward my mom. We sat and watched my dad die from cancer six years ago. *What is she thinking? I am worried about her. Is she thinking I am going to die too?* If she was worried, she didn't show it. She seemed as tough as nails. I didn't want to go there now. We had things to do.

Before the surgeon came in, we wrote down some questions, so we were somewhat prepared. We decided it was time to tell Kristen.

"Hi, Kris," Mom greeted with a shaky voice.

"Hey, Mom. How's it going?"

Mom came out and said it, "Not so good. We got the results of the CT scan. Vicki has two tumors in her chest. They think it is some form of lymphoma or thymoma. They want to do a biopsy tomorrow."

The phone went silent. It seemed like minutes went by. Kristen was trying to gain her composure.

"Um…wow. Okay. I am so sorry. I am going to find a flight to be there with you guys."

She said she would spend the rest of the evening packing and researching lymphoma so we would have the information after the surgery.

Dr. Liptay, the thoracic surgeon, walked in. Once again, I was surprised at the doctor's age. He was tall, handsome, confident, and sympathetic. Again, I searched for a wedding ring. None. Good. Even in my shocked state, I was checking out the doctors.

Anyway, Dr. Liptay made me feel good about the surgery tomorrow. It was going to be somewhere between one and three in the afternoon.

"Which kind of cancer should I hope I have?" I asked.

"They are all treatable," he answered.

That did not tell me much, but I suppose it was the best thing to say. Apparently, doctors seemed to say things were treatable, but not curable. That's all I have heard so far. We shook hands and said we would see each other tomorrow.

My mom and I decided to pick a friend and tell them about the cancer and have them call other friends. I picked Julie. I picked Julie because she was a social worker who had dealt with terminal illness (not that I thought this was terminal) and knew most of my friends. She would find a good way to tell people.

I found that it was extremely hard to tell Julie. It was very hard to come out and tell someone you cared about that you have cancer. It was such a bad word.

I blurted it out, "Hi, Julie. Can you get a piece of paper? I want you to write something down for me." I paused. "I have cancer. Two tumors in my chest. They think that it is lymphoma—Hodgkin's lymphoma, non-Hodgkin's lymphoma, or thymoma. Write that down. I am going to have a biopsy tomorrow to figure out which kind it is."

I guess that was kind of similar to what Dr. Zaacks said to me, but I found it so hard to get out of my mouth. I think Julie was in shock also. She asked me a few questions, and I gave her a list of people to call. I told her that I didn't want anyone to call me that night, but they could call in the morning before my surgery. Julie said that she loved me and would pray for me.

After my mom left, I received two phone calls. Just the two people I wanted to talk to—to comfort me the night before surgery, Kristen and Heather. Even though Julie gave everyone instructions not to call me, that was not going to stop Heather. She called to support me and told me that she and Kurt wanted to be with me tomorrow. I cried. She was such a terrific friend. Heather said she would pick Kristen up at the airport and come straight to the hospital. They should arrive right around when the surgery was supposed to take place. I talked to Kurt for a while, and we were all set for the next day. I was glad to have Heather and Kurt there for me. They were super supportive, just like when my dad was dying from cancer. They were always there for me.

I had a hard time getting to sleep, thinking about cancer and surgery and all. I tried to keep my thoughts off of it by watching Nick at Nite again, but it was difficult not to think about things. I prayed and finally fell asleep. Again, I had my sheets and gown changed like a kid who wets their bed. I put a towel around my wet hair. *I am not enjoying these new symptoms!*

May 25, 2000

Once again, I woke up bright and early. Today was a big day. I was not allowed to eat. I had the usual doctor and nurse visits and sat around waiting. My mom came and waited with me. Time went by so slowly. That was the slowest morning of my life. Finally around 1:00 p.m., they took me down for surgery. I was so relieved to be getting it over with.

They brought my mom and me to the same prep room that I went to for the muscle and nerve biopsy. I was lying on a bed with curtains on either side of me. There was a woman to my right who had just been given her anesthesia medication. On the other side of me was a man getting ready for a knee operation. While we were waiting, my mom and I listened to the woman next to us.

"This is great. I feel great. I love drugs—all kinds of drugs. I love marijuana. I love cocaine. I love all drugs." My mom and I giggled.

The anesthesiologist walked in. "Are you doing these drugs now?"

"Oh no. I haven't had marijuana or cocaine in fifteen years, but I love them."

That started my mom off. She said, "Vicki, they're going to ask you if you've done drugs before, and you have to tell the truth."

I laughed. This was the last thing I was worried about at this point. I highly doubted if the doctor was going to start questioning me on my drug habits. "Don't worry, Mom, they're not going to ask me, and if they do, I will tell the truth. I don't do drugs."

Then, they started the IV medications. I do not remember much of this part. I remember my mom telling me that I was not acting like myself. I asked her who or what I was acting like. She said, "I don't know, but you are not acting like yourself."

I remember wondering what was different about me. From what I found out later, I talked to anyone who would listen to me in the prep room. I tried to talk to anyone who walked by. I told everyone what a great time my mom and I had in Barbados. "I **love** Barbados!" I do not remember this, but according to my mom, I told the whole place how wonderful Barbados is.

The last thing I remember before my surgery was being wheeled into the operating room and hearing the doors bang open. My sister came running into the room yelling, "I'm here!"

Before I passed out, I had this vision of my sister's smiling face in my face. I will never forget that vision because it was the first thing I remembered when I came to in the recovery room. I thought to myself, as I remembered seeing her face, *Kristen must be here.*

The next thing I remembered was a phone call in the recovery room. It was Julie. Somehow she figured out how to call the recovery room at the exact time I was waking up. The nurse told her I was doing fine. It was then that Dr. Liptay walked in. I was still out of it. I looked up at the handsome doctor and thought, *what a nice vision!*

I asked, "Am I okay?"

"Yes, the surgery was a success and you are fine."

"What do I have?" I asked.

"You have some sort of lymphoma—either Hodgkin's or non-Hodgkin's. I'm not sure yet. It is not thymoma."

Then, I passed out.

I came to again back in my room. I think. Everything was so blurry. My mom, Kristen, Heather, and Kurt were sitting in the room waiting for me. I do not remember what we talked about, but I do know that the chest tube sticking out of my chest was making it very hard to breathe. Each breath I took hurt. Soon everyone left the room and I was left trying to breathe. I was up all night asking for drugs. I could not sleep due to the chest-tube pain. I didn't even notice if I had night sweats or not. One of the nurses warned me to get painkillers for when they take out the tube the next day. She said it really hurts when they yank the tube out. *Good, one more thing to look forward to.*

I must have drifted off around 4:00 a.m. Around 5:30 a.m., the door slowly opened in my room. I looked up to see Kurt standing there with some orange juice and a muffin. He bent over to kiss me and wished me well. I grinned at him and barely got out a whisper to thank him. He told me to go back to sleep. He went off to work. I fell back to sleep with a smile on my face thinking, *I have some really super friends.*

May 26, 2000

I woke up feeling like I had been in a car accident. I do not know what that feels like, but I felt all beat up, like I was in a brawl. I still couldn't breathe very well. All I wanted was to get the damn tube out of me. After Kurt came with food and juice, Kristen came by with more food for me. I did not want any food. I wanted the damn tube out of me. I asked every nurse or doctor who came in the room, "Can I have this tube taken out?" They all said, "In a while." *How long is a while?*

I checked my bed in the morning. No night sweats. I contemplated night sweats. Obviously, some mysterious thing happens once you fall asleep. Once you hit REM or something, the sweat must come pouring out of you somehow. *What triggers it?* The lack of night sweats probably meant that I never really had a good sleep. I needed to research this night-sweat phenomena. I needed to get the human library on this one, when we had a chance.

A doctor came by and told me that I could be discharged today. I thought they were nuts. I couldn't walk and I had this damn tube in me. I felt worse than I had felt the whole week I had been in the hospital. I was kind of used to the hovering in the hospital. I did not want to go home. I was scared to go home and fight the cancer battle. I had such a long road to travel before I was going to be well, I assumed.

They finally came by to take the tube out around noon. Kristen made sure they gave me medication for the pain. *That sister of mine is very assertive. When she wants something done, she makes sure it gets done.* They wiggled it around for a while and then yanked the tube out. It did not hurt nearly as bad as I thought, but I was shocked to see how long the tube was. It looked like there was a foot and a half inside me. *Where the heck did the tube fit? I already have a couple of tumors in my chest, how did a foot and a half of tubing fit in there as well?* Oh well, the damn tube was out.

The doctor called and told me the preliminary biopsy results were back and it looked like I had Hodgkin's lymphoma. I was a bit spaced out on drugs and was not really prepared for this conversation. I said, "Okay." He told me that Hodgkin's was a very treatable cancer. I was lucky. He started spewing more information that I did not comprehend. I did hear that the chemotherapy treatment was going to be harsh. Hmmmmm…

I stopped him, "Listen, I am all jammed up on painkillers. Can you please talk to my sister?"

I handed her the phone, and she proceeded to ask a bunch of questions and scribble down some notes.

I finally know what I have! The doctor had given us the name of an oncologist and made an appointment for the following week. He said she was top-notch. Kristen had all the details. I was ready to meet my oncologist. I had cancer and was going to have to have the dreaded chemo or radiation or something awful. It was supposed to be harsh. I had to get myself psychologically ready for this. I wanted to take a nap. Kristen left.

I slept great without the tube in me. I had a nice dark room on a beautiful sunny day. The door slowly opening awakened me. It was Heather. She put a present down on the bed and tried to sneak out. I wouldn't let her leave. I opened the gift with her. It was a little four-inch Waterford crystal angel. It was beautiful. It instantly became a symbol to me. The angel still sits on my nightstand today.

It watches over me, protects me, and has gotten me through a lot. Little did she know what a wonderful gift that was. We chatted for a while. I updated her on the Hodgkin's diagnosis and my new oncologist. *What great friends I have!*

In the afternoon, the doctor came by to see if I was ready to be discharged. He inspected my incisions, and I tried to walk for him. I told him that I really was not ready to leave. He agreed.

Kristen and Mom came by before they went out to dinner. They brought a bottle of wine to celebrate. *Are you allowed to do that?* I didn't know what we were celebrating. I had cancer. *Maybe we are celebrating getting out of the hospital? Maybe we are celebrating the fact that I know what I have? Maybe we are celebrating the fact that Hodgkin's is highly treatable?* I didn't care what we were celebrating; the wine was nice. *Typical of Mom to bring wine to a hospital. What a nut!* A couple glasses of wine and a good night's sleep were exactly what I needed.

May 27, 2000

I was discharged and moved to my mom's couch. I was really sore from the surgeries. I was mostly sore from the thoracic surgery, but the muscle and nerve biopsy made it hard to walk. When I turned my foot in a certain position, shocks ran through my foot and leg. The chunk of muscle missing from my leg made it hard to put much weight on my foot.

I had Vicodin to take to deal with the pain. After taking the first dose, I received a fifteen-minute lecture from my mom on how it is extremely addictive and not to take too much. I had never taken Vicodin before to my knowledge but didn't think I was going to become addicted from one non-refillable prescription. I shared this feeling with her. She proceeded to name famous celebrities who had become addicted to painkillers. I argued that the celebrities had more than one prescription to become addicted, but there was no winning. I had to sneak Vicodin when I felt like I needed it. *That made me feel like an addict. Maybe I am one?*

The human library had looked up all kinds of information on Hodgkin's lymphoma. We sat around reading all of this information from the internet and prepared a list of questions for the oncologist. The more I read, the more I got depressed, so I stopped reading. The medical information on the internet had a way of bringing out the worst cases. The treatment's side effects sounded just horrible. I figured I had anywhere from 50-90 percent survival rate. Earlier I was concentrating on the 90 percent survival rate, and now I was looking at the 50 percent survival rate. Half full/half empty. Apparently, the type of chemo that Hodgkin's patients have was supposed to be not just harsh but unbearable. That was when I stopped reading. We still needed to get the type and stage of Hodgkin's to determine the treatment and survival rate. I decided to put together my list of questions and try not to think about it.

May 29, 2000

Memorial Day. Kristen, my mom, and I went to my dad's grave and planted flowers. I watched. It was a beautiful day and I was glad to be out. After saying prayers, we went downtown to plant flowers in my garden in Lincoln Park. Again, I watched.

We dropped Kristen off at the airport. I was so glad that she had come to support me. This has been such a hard week on my mom also. We both needed Kristen. She was so assertive in the hospital.

She didn't accept no for an answer. I was sorry we didn't have such a great time for her visit, but sometimes you just have to do the things you have to do.

When she left, it was back to just my mom and me to tackle the oncologist and come up with a plan of attack. We felt pretty lost. We wanted to be so on top of it, but we felt like a couple of lost souls with a list of questions. Somehow this was different than when Dad was diagnosed. *Maybe it is because it is me? Maybe because I am younger? Maybe it is because he was so far along? I am not sure.*

When we got back to my mom's, I called my voicemail. I had a few calls from friends from my old job, my new job, and from Alan, Bill, and Christian. I decided to put the calls off until the next day. They were not discussions that I felt like having at the moment.

My night sweats started in the hospital and continued at home. The night sweats continued with a vengeance. I began to wear a bandana or towel at night to keep my head warm and put towels down on the mattress and pillow. I changed my nightshirt a few times a night. The whole night-sweat phenomena was annoying, but I started losing the weight I wanted to lose. *Bonus. My cup is half full. I am losing weight.*

Chapter Six

June 2000: My Plan

> "All you need is the plan, the road map, and the courage to press on to your destination."
>
> — Earl Nightingale

June 1, 2000

My millennium was supposed to be all about making positive changes in health, relationships, and career. My health diminished significantly. My relationships with men were going nowhere fast. My career had a positive outlook, if I could get over my health issues. I had to pivot and make an adjustment to my millennium goals. I decided to focus on #1 cancer and #2 start-up, for now. Ditch the men.

Today was a big day. I met with my oncologist, who was to become a huge part of my life. Kristen had done her research. She was a top-notch hematologist oncologist named Dr. Kim. *I guess that is a lymphoma doctor?* I was about to learn a whole new vocabulary.

Dr. Kim walked in and was very business-like. Mom and I were so anxious to ask our questions that we could barely contain ourselves. She had to slow us down. She had a speech she wanted to get through, and we weren't letting her. She explained as much as she could about the plan—*my plan*. I guess there is a gold standard for Hodgkin's lymphoma that people take: ABVD (Adriamycin, Bleomycin, Vinblastine, Decacarbazine) chemotherapy for six or eight months, every other week. *I do this and I get better. Okay, that's my plan. Let's do this!*

Not so fast. I had more tests to do before I could start the chemotherapy. I needed a bone marrow biopsy to see if cancer has spread to my bone marrow. I also needed a slew of tests to represent a baseline for "before" chemotherapy. I needed a gallium scan, pulmonary function test, more blood tests, etc. I was tired of tests but glad to know I had a plan! This illness had been so frustrating trying to figure out what to do, and now, I finally had a plan! My plan! It almost made me feel better knowing I had a plan.

I told the oncologist about all of the weakness, throbbing, and numbness in my extremities, and she didn't seem to care. This bothered me. It was obviously related to the cancer, but she would not confirm it. I also told her about the night sweats and fatigue, which were classic symptoms of Hodgkin's lymphoma. She said those symptoms should go away with the chemotherapy.

The big question was about my hair. I had a feeling I was going to lose it, and she confirmed it. I was okay with that. I know other people would be really upset about losing their hair, but I figured, if that's part of the plan, then bring it on. I just wanted to kill the cancer and get better. My hair would grow out eventually.

We finished asking our questions, which took about an hour and a half. I didn't care if other patients had to wait. I needed to understand "my plan." My plan was going to keep me alive and feeling better. It took so long and so many doctor visits to get here, and I was going to make sure we were thorough.

June 2, 2000

I would like to forget today. Mom took me to the hospital for my bone marrow biopsy. This test would tell me information about what stage I was in, white and red blood cell count, and if lymphoma was in my bone marrow. I guess I needed to have the test, but I wasn't looking forward to it.

Dr. Kim assured me that the biopsy wasn't that difficult. With the local anesthetic, it was supposed to feel like some pressure on my hip. That was not the case. It was kind of like the EMG. I was not prepared for the pain.

She had me lie on my side and numbed my right hip bone. Okay, that didn't hurt too much. Then, she took out a long needle. I wish I didn't turn around to see it. I wish she had warned me. It was really, really long. I squeezed my mom's hand until she yelled at me to stop. At first, it didn't hurt bad, and then, I felt the pressure. Then, I felt excruciating pain as she grabbed a chunk of my hip bone. OUCH!! I was dripping with sweat and light-headed as I tried to gather myself together. *Wow! That hurts!*

After I gathered myself together, Mom took me to the gallium scan. It was a breeze as far as tests go. Gallium loves Hodgkin's. When you are injected with gallium, a radioactive medicine, it glows and lights up the tumors.

While I was at the hospital, I also had a pulmonary function test (PFT). Since I was going to the hospital, we wanted to get as much in as possible. Apparently, one of the ingredients in the chemo cocktail hurts your lungs, so the PFT was a baseline of sorts. It was an easy test in comparison with the others. The test consisted of blowing into a tube on and off for about twenty minutes. By the end, I was exhausted. It was a long day.

I had a hard time getting in and out of the car and sitting the rest of the day. It was tough when I went out to dinner with my mom's friend, Nancy. I sat down on my left butt cheek for the whole dinner. Actually, I didn't notice the pain that much, because the discussion was so engaging. Nancy was undergoing chemotherapy for breast cancer and shared her story and tips with me. Her chemo cocktail was different from mine, but a lot of what she shared applied. I asked a ton of questions and took a bunch of notes. After the butt bone biopsy, dinner made me feel better being in the company of someone who understood and cared about what I was about to go through.

Nancy told me, "You need to buy a journal and write down everything from how you are feeling before, during, and after chemo, to questions you have for each doctor's visit, to how much of each medication you should take. You will find it helpful in the future when you can't remember things. I get nervous for appointments and can't remember what questions to ask or what the answers are. It is always good to take your journal with you to appointments and procedures."

I was getting such good advice and was very thankful for her support. I went and bought a journal the next day.

June 3, 2000

I began writing in my new journal. I had a lot of information to document about my diagnosis, medications, and procedures. I wrote about my symptoms. I wrote about my hospital stay. I listed my medications, doses, side effects, doctors' names and numbers, diagnoses, chemo, dates, questions, etc. My journal became my diary, my bible, my dictionary, my calendar, and my prized possession. I didn't go anywhere without it.

Diagnosis:
Hodgkin's Stage IIB Nodular Sclerosis
Cardiophrenic tumor—4 x 10 cm (surrounding heart)
Mediastinal tumor—2 x 4 cm (mid-chest)
90% 5-year survival rate
80-85% curable
10-15% recurrence

Recommended Treatment:
ABVD
- *Adriamycin (damages heart, causes nausea, hair loss, fatigue, skin sensitivity, mouth sores, nickname—"Red Devil")*
- *Bleomycin (damages lungs)*
- *Vinblastine (causes neuropathy, hair loss, nausea, constipation)*
- *DTIC—Dacarbazine (causes fatigue, nausea, skin sensitivity, infections)*

WBC—needs to be 1500 for treatment

Medications:
- Prednisone
- Pepcid

- *Zofran*
- *Neurontin*
- *Lorazepam*
- *Compazine*
- *Sulfamethoxazole*
- *Centrum*
- *Tums*
- *Tylenol*
- *Celebrex*

After writing in my journal, I made a few phone calls. I had been putting off calling Alan back. "My plan" did not include him. *Sorry, Alan.* My plan didn't include men. I had to focus on my health and my job. I was in a different mindset. I decided I would keep up the relationship with Bill, because it was pretty platonic anyway. I had to ditch Alan though.

I got his answering machine!

"Hi, Alan. It's Vicki. Sorry it has taken me so long to call you back, but I haven't been myself since the diagnosis. I need to focus on my health and don't have time for a relationship. I'm sorry. It has been nice getting to know you. Take care!" I explained on his answering machine.

I got off easy. I know it is sort of rude to leave a message like that, but it is not like he was a boyfriend. We were just getting to know each other. If he were a boyfriend, I would have wanted to lean on him during my time of need. It wouldn't be awkward.

Next, I called Bill back and left a nice message. After that, I emailed Christian and gave him an update. Done. I am all caught up with my journal and my men.

June 6, 2000

They always say to get a second opinion. Dr. Kim told me that ABVD was the gold standard, so my treatment should have been straightforward, but I still thought it was a good idea to get a second opinion before I started treatment. Kristen did some research and determined that there was a very reputable hematologist oncologist at Northwestern Hospital downtown.

Today was the day for my second opinion. Northwestern Hospital was ginormous and made me feel intimidated. It was so easy to get lost wandering through all of the buildings, floors, and halls. I decided to get there an hour early in case I couldn't find the office. After getting lost a few times, I finally found the waiting room. It turned out, the room took up the entire floor of the building. I got off the elevator and the room was filled with cancer patients—maybe fifty or more. Lots of wheelchairs. Lots of skinny old people in hospital gowns. Lots of bandanas covering bald heads. Lots of depressed looking people sitting around waiting. Soon, I joined them and was one of them. My anxious mood quickly changed to depression. I brought all of my scans, doctors' notes, and journal to the appointment.

When my name was called, I jumped up, gathered my stuff, and followed the nurse back to a small room away from the enormous gloomy waiting room. My mood moved with me—back to anxiousness. The nurse proceeded to ask me all of the standard questions of what brings me there. I thought it was obvious.

The great oncologist came bursting into the room and spent all of ten minutes with me, never wanting to see my scans or tests. He suggested ABVD and left. I left the great gloomy Northwestern

Hospital feeling confident in my original decision to be treated in the cozy Glenbrook Hospital.

June 7, 2000

I was trying to regulate my steroid intake with Dr. Zaacks. I know that seems odd. It was like I was a bodybuilder trying to regulate steroid use, but I was really trying to manage the throbbing weakness in my extremities. I was trying to wean off of Prednisone. Every time I got on a low dose, my extremities got worse. I documented it in my journal—how much medication I was taking and how I was feeling. It was frustrating. The whole cancer situation wouldn't have been so bad if I didn't have these issues. None of the doctors knew how to deal with it either. There wasn't a gold standard for the numbness, throbbing, and weakness in my arms and legs. They didn't know what to do with me. Dr. Kim acted like I was a complainer and minimized the situation. That was annoying.

I tried to focus on work, but it was hard with all of my health issues going on. I finished up some of the proposals I was working on and made a few sales calls. I had bad timing with this new job, but I wanted to make it work. I worked late into the evening because I knew I would be useless the next day—my first chemo. Work kept me busy, so I didn't have to think about it too much. I slept really well too. I was so tired after working all day. Night sweats invaded me as I slept deeply. I woke up sopping wet twice during the night and changed my clothes and turban.

June 8, 2000

I woke up excited and nervous for my big day—*the start of my plan! Let's go!!*

Heather took me to the hospital at 8:00 a.m. to start the process. I had to get a portacath surgically implanted in my chest before I could start the treatment. I guess they decided that was the best way to give me the chemo, especially since my veins were so hard to poke. You can have chemotherapy and other medications and fluids delivered through a portacath. It is a small chamber or reservoir that sits under your skin at the end of your central line. I was told it was a four-inch tube into the artery in my neck.

Heather was with me while a radiologist surgeon operated. I was awake and talking the whole time. They gave me medications that made me loopy and unable to feel the surgery. Well, I didn't feel the pain, but I could feel the yanking of the tube through my chest under my skin. It was a very strange sensation.

Though I was pretty nervous to start, I was very loopy and chatty. I kept smiling at the handsome doctor. I tried to flirt with him and told him he was cute. Heather sat giggling in the corner. Then, I started giggling. The good doctor smiled and told me to hold still. *How many surgeries have I had in the last few weeks? I dunno...*

Why are all my surgeons so good-looking? Wow! Maybe I should have been a doctor instead of an engineer. Or maybe a nurse? Or maybe just work in a hospital?

Anyway, after I was ready to go with my new portacath, they wheeled me to the Kellogg Cancer Center for my treatment. My mom met us there, took over, and gave Heather a break from escorting me around the hospital.

Mom had worked that morning and was now available for the rest of my big day. Interestingly, she had been working at the hospital for the past few months as a volunteer greeter. Volunteering twice a week at the hospital for four hours was the first job she has had since she was twenty-four.

The Kellogg Cancer Center is where I met my nurse and new best friend, Daniela. Daniela gave me a large document to sign before chemo was to begin. I was still loopy from the surgery, so I wasn't quite sure what I was signing. The document described the possible side effects from the different ingredients to the chemo cocktail. It was terrifying to think that I could develop heart conditions, breast cancer, lung cancer, leukemia, infertility, osteoporosis, etc. from the chemo I was taking to save my life. My mom was even more terrified than I was. Probably because she was of the right mind.

"Daniela, am I reading this correctly? It says I can get all of these different kinds of cancer from taking the chemo that is supposed to get rid of my cancer? That doesn't make sense to me."

"Legally, we have to tell you about all of the **possible** long-term side effects of the chemo. The chances are slim of you getting any of them," she told us.

Daniela first tested the individual ingredients to the chemo cocktail on me to see if there were any adverse reactions. After I passed with flying colors, the chemo drip commenced. IV bag after IV bag dripped into my new portacath. I was ever so slowly being poisoned. All I really noticed was that Adriamycin was bright red, and the last one was a downer. I sat there watching TV for four hours.

When I say the last one was a downer, I mean, it was a **real** downer. As I watched TV, I suddenly started to cry. Mom looked up from her book and asked me, "What are you crying about?"

"I don't know," I replied.

"Well, stop," she uttered.

"I can't," I mumbled.

And on and on, I cried. At the end of the chemo, I stopped crying, and Mom took me to her house. I slept for about twelve hours. *I guess I needed it. Not a bad day, all in all.*

June 9, 2000

I woke up well rested. I didn't feel any different, except that I was sore from the portacath. I was still sweaty. My hair was still there. I was still weak with throbbing extremities. I didn't feel nauseous. I guess chemo doesn't work that fast. I thought about the day yesterday and documented it in my journal. Some of the day was foggy. I couldn't remember that much of the chemo. I wondered if that was normal. I drove home from Mom's house.

I had a strong desire to talk to people with Hodgkin's. The only information I had on the disease was what I found on the internet and what my doctors told me. I wanted to hear firsthand what it was going to be like to fight the battle.

Gilda's Club was right down the street from me, so I thought I would start there. Gilda Radner, from *Saturday Night Live*, passed away from ovarian cancer about ten years ago. Gilda's Club was created to help provide support to cancer patients like me. The office was located just a few blocks away from Second City on Wells Street, where she got her start. I walked down the street and found the door locked. There were no hours listed on the door. My search for support didn't start out very well. I took down the phone number and called when I got back home.

Gilda's Club was no help. *Maybe they are just starting out?* They didn't have anyone in their database who had Hodgkin's. Geez, I didn't know Hodgkin's was so unusual. They had lots of people in their database with breast, lung, and colon cancer, but not Hodgkin's.

I continued my search to the Cancer Wellness Center in Northbrook. They had all kinds of services available to cancer patients. They took down my information and told me they would call me back. In addition to finding someone with Hodgkin's to talk to, I was interested in support groups, informational sessions, and yoga. I signed up for a support group meeting. I started to feel better about my search for help.

June 10, 2000

I woke up in my own bed feeling well rested. My night sweats continued, but I only changed clothes once during the night. That was a start. I decided to get on the scale.

YIPPEE!!! I lost the ten pounds that I was determined to lose at the beginning of the year! Actually, I was down twelve pounds! Those night sweats must have done the trick! I guess I achieved one of my goals. I didn't like the way it happened, but it was a win. *I have to have something to be happy about, don't I?*

I didn't do too much today, because I wanted to save my energy for the evening. My arms and legs were throbbing from weaning off of Prednisone. My chest with the portacath was sore. I felt pretty beaten up from being cut up (ankle muscle and nerve biopsy, thoracic surgery for cancer biopsy, bone marrow biopsy, and portacath implant), but I felt like I should do something with myself. I went on a short walk to get outside and stretch my legs. It was a beautiful day. My neighborhood in Lincoln Park was so fun to walk around. There was always an exciting vibe in the air.

I was a block into my journey when I bumped into my friend Liz, who bowled me over with a big hug. "Vicki, it is so good to see you walking around! I have been thinking about you nonstop! How are you doing? How are you feeling?"

I worked with Liz at the corporation. She was in sales and had the personality for it. Always smiling and having a ball. It was obvious that news had spread about my cancer. I wasn't used to talking about it though.

"I am okay. I am feeling kind of tired though. I had my first chemo and it went well. I feel like a pin cushion from being poked and sliced. How are you doing?" I replied.

"Same as always. Trying to sell something. We all miss you at the corporation. We were all shocked at the news. Are you working?" she asked.

"Trying to, but it isn't easy. The start-up is very accommodating though," I responded.

Then Liz started to ask me about my cancer, "How do you get Hodgkin's lymphoma? Is it hereditary?"

"They don't really know. It isn't supposed to be hereditary."

"Do you think you got it from stress? I bet you, the job stress brought it on. I heard you can get cancer from stress. I have some books at home that might help you," she remarked.

What? Is she implying that I gave myself cancer from stress? What the hell?

I was dumbfounded. I didn't know how to respond. I think she was trying to help, but *really?*

"Sure. That would be nice. Well, gotta go!"

I had hoped that this wasn't the first of many people trying to tell me I gave myself Hodgkin's. I pondered it for the rest of my walk.

That night I went to the club to meet Heather and Kurt for dinner. It was my first real night out. I was tired, but okay. I walked into the bar to hugs and kisses. Everyone was so friendly. It was good to see friendly faces. No one tried to tell me I gave myself cancer. Although, it was kind of strange. I felt like I had a big "C" on my forehead and there was a spotlight on me. Everyone was friendly, but different. Some people, I hardly knew, came up to talk to me to let me know how sorry they were. Then, some good friends avoided me like I was a leper. Very strange. I guess people just don't know what to say or do. Avoidance is not the way to go though.

Dinner was exhausting, but it was great being out. I enjoyed hearing about Heather and Kurt's kids. They were so adorable. I loved being Aunt Vicki. Besides Kirby, they were the closest thing I had to having kids. I made a mental note to go for a visit soon. They really cheered me up!

June 15, 2000

Mom's friend, Nancy, told me to go to Jerome Krause to buy my wig. Insurance would cover it. She also told me to go before my hair started falling out. So, that's what I did.

Rita was a hoot. She was a boisterous woman who commanded Jerome Krause. Apparently, all of the cancer-afflicted ladies on the North Shore went to see Rita. She was practically a celebrity. As we spoke, I checked out her hair, wondering if it was a wig. If it was a wig, it was a damn good one. Her hair was all made up, and she had tons of makeup on.

Since I already had short hair, Rita told me it would be easier. Dealing with my hair falling out would be a breeze. She was very knowledgeable about hair loss from chemo and shared that knowledge with me. She asked me a ton of questions. Do I want the same length? Do I want the same color? Do I want the same style? Do I want the same thickness? I started to panic. I didn't know what I wanted. I started to think about it. *If I am going to change my hair, this is a good time to do it. I could go long blonde. I could go curly or straight. I could go with something totally different, and then change it if I don't like it.* This was my chance to have any hair style I wanted!

I decided to have Rita match my hair as close as possible to my real hair. I guess I was a chicken. My wig was going to be ready in two weeks. I hoped my hair didn't fall out before then.

After my wig appointment, I went to see Dr. Liptay to get my stitches out. I had three incisions, but only one with real stitches. The other two had glue. I am not sure why they close you up using different means, but they do. I was excited to see Dr. Liptay, because he was so handsome and nice. I enjoyed being around him.

Dr. Liptay came into the room and shook my hand. "How are you doing, Vicki?"

"Okay, I guess. I had my first chemo and am feeling okay," I responded.

"One down! You are on your way! Let's look at these incisions," he said while inspecting my beat-up chest. "They look fantastic! Now, let's get these stitches out."

He seemed like he was in a good mood and wanted to talk while he was working on me. "Your friend Julie stops by every once in a while to check up on you. Did you know that she called the recovery room while you were in surgery to check on how you were doing? She must really care about you. She certainly knows her way around a hospital."

I chuckled. "Yes. I don't remember it well, but a nurse told me she was on the phone in the recovery room. Yes, she is a great friend."

Julie did care a lot. She worked at the hospital and knew her way around. She was very assertive. She was right there when Heather had her babies (or not far away). Thinking about Julie gave me a warm feeling inside and made me smile.

That evening, I went to my first support group meeting at the Cancer Wellness Center. I didn't know what to expect, but I was looking forward to it. *Maybe I will meet someone with Hodgkin's?*

There was a circle of about twelve chairs set up in the room with some people milling around drinking coffee and eating cookies. I felt like I was walking into an AA meeting. Not that I had been to an AA meeting, but the room looked like what I'd seen on TV. I had never been to a support group and didn't know what to expect. I introduced myself to a few people, and we all sat down.

A guy in his 40s introduced himself as Jeremy and kicked off the session. He was a colon cancer survivor volunteer. Jeremy asked us all to introduce ourselves and share a little bit about ourselves. I was so glad I didn't go first. I wasn't sure what to share. I listened intently as people told their stories. People asked questions here and there.

I was the youngest one there. People ranged from forty-ish to eighty-ish years old. They were wearing all kinds of different clothes from very casual to suits. No one looked sick. I still felt like I was at an AA meeting.

"Hi, I'm Vicki, and I was diagnosed three weeks ago with Hodgkin's lymphoma," I started out. "It is my first meeting. I am here to see if I can connect with other Hodgkin's patients. Does anyone have Hodgkin's?"

I looked around the room, and everyone shook their heads. *Oh well...I tried.* I went on to describe my experience, and people gave me suggestions on what to do about my extremities.

"Try biofeedback."

"Try meditation."

"Try yoga."

"That's just the chemo giving you neuropathy."

"Try acupuncture."

"Get a massage."

"Go to a chiropractor."

UGH! So many natural healing methods to try when I am looking for the gold standard—a golden nugget. I just want a pill to make it go away.

I smiled, thanked them, and wrote down their suggestions in my journal.

I went home thinking I was never going to find anyone with Hodgkin's to talk to. There was no one in the support group, and they hadn't called me to give me the name of someone from their database either. I thought about the support group. I guess it was helpful to talk to people with cancer. They did give me some tips to follow up on, but I was not sure if I was going to run back there anytime soon. *I'll put it on the back burner for now.*

June 17, 2000

I had a relaxing day today, because I had plans that night. I never wanted to do too much during the day when I had plans to go out. I did a little work and took a short walk. No one told me this, but I thought it was a good idea to take walks. I did a lot of sitting around with my legs elevated. My ankles and legs felt much better elevated. The worst position was having my legs hang down. I had a hard time walking after they hung down for a long period of time. Walking helped me mentally and physically.

My amazing friends Margie and Hugh had me over for dinner. Hugh was Heather's older brother and like a brother to me. Just like in *Caddyshack*, in high school, Hugh caddied at Skokie Country Club and dated Margie who was a waitress. Kindhearted Margie was a terrific addition to the family.

They also invited Hugh's and Heather's parents and my mom for dinner. It was a fun dinner party set at their long dining room table, which was decorated beautifully. Margie went all out. Their table was set with fine china, silver, and crystal. Margie and Hugh were excellent entertainers and cooks. They were serving Silver Oak cabernet and Grgich chardonnay with the meal. I loved wine. Grgich was one of my favorites. I had not had any wine since I started chemo. I made a note to address that with Dr. Kim. I didn't have any wine that night but added wine to my list of questions for my next visit. Eight months was a long time to abstain from chardonnay.

The dinner may have sounded formal but was quite informal. We were all such good friends. Our two families went on a number of vacations together while we were growing up. We went on ski vacations in Wisconsin, Michigan, Colorado, and Utah. We were all pretty athletic people—skiing, golf, and tennis. In addition, there were no shrinking violets in the group.

As the guest of honor, I was at the head of the table. My mom was to my right, and Heather and Hugh's dad, Hodie, to my left. It was a four-course meal, so we had a lot of time to catch up. I was the major attraction at the table. I had to be on. I was glad that I rested most of the day.

Margie was pretty much all caught up with my diagnosis and "my plan," but the others had a lot of questions, especially my dinner partner, Hodie, who was quite the personality. The kids had nicknamed him "The General." With his big personality, almost every time Hodie spoke to me, he whacked me on the arm with the back of his hand.

Whack. "So, Vicki, how is the chemo going so far?"

Whack. "How was the hospital food?"

Whack. "You should come up to the lake house and relax."

Finally, Margie jumped in, "Hodie! Stop hitting Vicki!"

Thank you, Margie! I had a fantastic time but was starting to feel beat up.

That night I slept well. I barely had any night sweats. *Hurray! Maybe the night sweats are ending? Maybe the chemo is working?* This was very good news. I got on the scale. More good news! I dropped sixteen pounds since the beginning of the year. My cup was more than half full!

June 22, 2000

Today I had my second chemo. My plan included having chemo every two weeks for six to eight months. After six months, they were supposed to check my CT scan again to see if I needed more chemo. I was really hoping to be done in six months. Then, I could have a celebratory Christmas. I figured, if I do everything they tell me, I should be done in six months. That's the way it should work. *Right?*

My cousin Sharon took me to my second chemo. I didn't know this at the time, but there was a whole process I would follow for each chemo. The first time was different, because of the whole portacath implant procedure. We got to the Kellogg Cancer Center at Glenbrook Hospital at about 8:30 a.m. to check in, and they sent me to the lab for a complete blood count (CBC) blood test. I was told I could not have chemo if my white blood count (WBC) was less than 1,500. A low WBC means that you do not have enough white blood cells to fight off infection. I got the test done and went back to the small waiting room.

Sharon and I hung out until they got the results back—about an hour. It was a good time to catch up with Sharon. She and her brothers and sisters were very close cousins to my small family. Since my sister lived in California, Sharon became like a sister to me. She was such a sweetheart. It felt good sharing my cancer journey with her. She was happy to be a part of my journey.

I felt like a lot of friends and family wanted to help along the way. Bringing me to chemo was one of the ways they could help. My chemo nurse, Daniela, called us into my personal chemo room, which consisted of a recliner chair, a bed, two regular chairs, and a TV. I sat in the recliner chair. I must have passed the WBC test, or I wouldn't be moving forward with the chemo. I introduced Sharon to Daniela. I was informed that my WBC was 1,400. My heart sank.

"So…does that mean I can't have chemo today?" I inquired.

"Dr. Kim said that we can have the chemo, but she ordered a few things to be added to it," Daniela replied.

"Like, what kind of things?" I asked, hesitantly.

"Just a few additional medications to keep you from having an infection."

I guess 1,400 wasn't too low. A normal WBC is between 4,000 and 11,000. A WBC of 1,400 seems pretty low to me. I didn't ask any more questions, because I didn't want to skip chemo. *Let's get this done!*

The chemo treatment commenced with a stab into my port. It took about four hours. This was the order of medications:

- Zofran

- Tylenol
- Benadryl
- Saline solution
- Decadron
- DTIC–2 hours
- Vinblastine
- Adriamycin
- Bleomycin
- Steroids–500mg

The DTIC made me really tired, and the steroids kept me awake. I am not sure what was supposed to keep me from infection, but I was okay not knowing. I was also supposed to drink a lot of water. I took notes in my journal.

I didn't cry this time, but I did fall asleep. Sharon just kept watching the movie. I think she left the room for a while, because she was eating a sandwich and drinking Diet Coke when I woke up. I wasn't sure what was going on in the movie, but it wasn't over.

"I'm so sorry I fell asleep!" I told her.

"No problem. I was hungry and got a sandwich. They changed your IV and brought you lunch, if you are hungry," she said as she pulled over the lunch tray. The food actually looked inviting: grilled ham and cheese, fries, fruit.

"Yum. I am kind of hungry." Sharon proceeded to catch me up on the movie as I ate. I was almost finished with the chemo poisoning, and the steroids started kicking in.

My limbs felt better as we walked to the car. I think the steroids were helping. I was on a high of sorts. It felt good. I thanked Sharon for taking me as she dropped me off at Mom's house. It was not a bad chemo day. I felt good and had a nice time with Sharon. *What more could I ask for?*

I spent the night at Mom's on chemo days. It was just easier that way. I wasn't sure how I was going to respond and felt better being around her. Mom bought a townhouse after Dad died. It was decorated nicely with art and furniture from our old house. She still had my old bedroom furniture, including my old desk in the guest bedroom. As I stayed there more and more, I started filling the drawers and closet. It became my room again.

That night, my mom asked me if she could plan some trips for us to get out of town between treatments. That idea perked me up.

"Where do you want to go?" I asked her.

"Oh, I don't know. Maybe Italy? Maybe the Caribbean? How about Barbados? I want to take you away from all of this. It is pretty depressing. Wouldn't the treatment be easier on you if you were lying on the beach? I want to do something special for you. I don't want this year to be all negative. We could have some fun!" Mom threw out.

"I imagine so, but that sounds pretty expensive."

"Don't worry. I have it covered. I have some money saved for a rainy day, and *this* is a rainy day," she said. "In fact, it seems like it is pouring. We'll have to do both Italy and the Caribbean."

Does she think I am dying? I wasn't sure. *Is that why she wants to go on trips with me?* I thought I would ask Kristen what she thought on the topic.

I had a wonderful night's sleep. I thought about Italy and Barbados. It sounded amazing. I hoped that we actually went through with it.

June 23, 2000

I woke up and analyzed how I felt. I did that a lot these days. I was trying to figure out my schedule. I was trying to figure out when I was at my best and my worst. I wrote it all down in my journal. I think the steroids kept me up for a while, but I also had some meds that made me sleep. All in all, I had a pretty good night's sleep. My extremities were doing okay too. I started wearing the hospital leggings to sleep to help my poor numb, tingling, throbbing legs. I started wearing them around the house too. No one told me to do it, but I think they helped. Mom thought I looked stupid in them, but I didn't care.

I started feeling spacey. I felt spacey all of the time. I felt like an airhead. I felt like a dumb blonde. I started becoming forgetful. I took notes in my journal and thought I would ask the doctor about it. I assumed this was from the chemo, but I don't remember that being a side effect. Later, I found out that the feeling was called "chemo brain." *Yes, I have chemo brain.*

In addition to the issues with my extremities, my neck and face blew up like a balloon. They were so swollen, I could barely recognize myself. It was strange because I lost a bunch of weight and still looked fat. In the past, when I lost weight, my face always looked skinnier. It was fatter than ever.

I drove home that morning, back down to my townhouse. Lately, I had problems driving when my extremities were bad. That day, I started out amazingly well and went downhill from there as I came off of the steroid high. That afternoon, the throbbing commenced and I was miserable. I was supposed to go out with Cate and Julie that night and had to cancel for a date with my TV and the couch. I was watching TV a lot. Ever since I was in the hospital, I couldn't focus on much more than TV, magazines, and some forced concentration on the start-up. Even that was becoming more difficult to do.

My answering machine had five calls on it from Alan, Bill, Heather, Julie, and the Cancer Wellness Center. I was so excited! The Cancer Wellness Center had a Hodgkin's cancer survivor for me to talk to! They gave me the name of a guy who was a five-year Hodgkin's cancer survivor. I couldn't wait to call him in the morning. The others would have to wait.

June 24, 2000

I analyzed my health and journaled it. Hands/arms—slightly throbbing. Feet/legs—throbbing. Left ankle—really throbbing. Spacey. Tired. No nausea. No loss of hair (based on pillow check). I took my meds and started my day.

I called Jeff, the survivor, at 9:00 a.m. I got his answering machine. *Damn!* I left a message. I worked for a few hours and called it a day. My work days were getting shorter, as I could only focus for short periods of time. I was starting to feel guilty about the effort I was putting into my new job. I wondered what they thought about me and my cancer. I bet they wished they had hired someone else to be in charge of sales for the start-up. I would have to talk to Marc about it. I didn't want to be the reason that the start-up was unsuccessful. I really believed in the company and our vision. I went on a walk. My walks were getting shorter too.

I was awakened from a nap by the phone. It was Jeff. We spoke for a half an hour.

"Hi, Vicki. This is Jeff. I got your message. They told me that you would be calling. Thanks for calling," he began.

"Hi, Jeff. Thank *you* for calling *me*! I have so many questions for you. I don't know where to begin."

"That's okay. Let me tell you a little about myself," he continued. "I am forty years old and was diagnosed in 1995. I had ABVD for six months. It was tough, but it got rid of the tumor in my neck. I was pretty sick but made a full recovery within about a year or so. I actually did a marathon last year."

Wow! He did a marathon after Hodgkin's and ABVD! I was elated to hear this news! AND, he had six months, not eight months, of chemo! I was so happy! I proceeded to ask him all of my questions and got to know Jeff a little better. I was excited to have this new friend. Of course, I think I got a little too excited. My mind was racing. I knew I had put men on the back burner, but I was still a little boy crazy. Every guy I met at a certain age range was a possibility. I was brought down to earth when told me he was married.

Knowing about Jeff, the marathon man, my outlook on cancer improved. I didn't think I would run a marathon but thought I could get back in shape after the treatment. Jeff and I agreed to keep in touch and maybe do lunch sometime. I called my mom to let her know about the conversation.

Chapter Seven

July 2000: My Move to Mom's

> "It is during our darkest moments that we must focus to see the light." — Aristotle

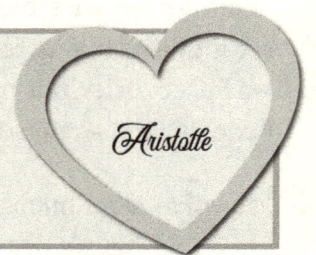

July 1, 2000

I analyzed my health, journaled, and packed up for a jaunt to Heather's family cottage. I went up there often for summertime fun. I loved water sports. I loved water skiing as much as snow skiing. There wouldn't be any water skiing this visit, but some good pontoon rides, swimming with noodles, and sun.

Heather asked me if I wanted a ride up to the cottage. I thought my legs and ankles were good enough to drive, so I did. On my way up to the cottage, I stopped at a farm stand on the side of the road and bought some tomatoes. I didn't want to come empty-handed. Then, I stopped for a few bottles of chardonnay. During my last chemo, I was told that I could have wine, but don't overdo it. Apparently, Adriamycin is not good for your heart, but I could have wine in limited quantities. I was excited to have some wine with my dinner.

After an hour and a half, I finally got to the lake house. The clan was all there and ready to go out on Hodie's pontoon boat. Heather, Kurt, Margie, Hugh, their parents, and kids were all there for the July 4th weekend. I was, once again, the highly esteemed guest of honor.

It was a gorgeous day on the lake. There wasn't a cloud in the sky. The waves were calm, almost like glass. I wished I could ski. It was the perfect day for it. I sat on the end of the dock with Heather's mom, Pam. Pam was a close friend of my mom's and a total hoot. I enjoyed sitting in the Adirondack chair chatting with her.

I whipped out the sunscreen. I was told that the chemo would make me burn easily, so I came prepared with my 50 SPF. I started lathering it on. About five minutes later, I was still lathering it on, when Pam started laughing.

"Vicki, I think you have put on enough sunscreen! You look like a ghost with all of that sunscreen on!"

"Well, they told me to be careful with the sun. I don't want to get fried," I replied.

"I don't think anything could get through *that* coating!" she exclaimed.

Okay, so maybe I overdid the sunscreen. I was just trying to do what I was told.

We had a marvelous day on the lake with the kids. I took a quick nap before dinner and woke up to a bustling group. Hugh and Kurt were out back grilling steaks, while Heather and Margie were helping Pam in the kitchen. Hodie came in from fishing with two of the kids. I helped set the table. As I set the table, I started thinking, *where is Hodie going to sit? I don't want to get bruised up again.* I put my glass of wine down at a spot in the middle of the table. I thought I would be safe there.

I was right. Hodie sat at one end and Pam sat at the other. I was safe! I helped pour the wine. We had my chardonnay and a cabernet. Everything seemed to be going fine until halfway through the dinner. Hodie belted out, "Who bought this rot-gut chardonnay?"

I slipped down in my seat as I looked around.

I caught Pam's eye, as she announced, "Vicki brought the chardonnay. Wasn't that nice of her?"

"Ugh. It's awful! Maybe it is just a bad bottle."

"Sorry," I winced.

I was so embarrassed. I should have bought a nicer bottle. *What have I done?*

Pam continued, "Don't worry. I have some good chardonnay in the fridge."

Pam jumped up, grabbed the bottles of wine on the table, and replaced them with a delicious chardonnay. At least my tomatoes were good. Everyone loved them.

July 2, 2000

I woke up to the clan running around at 9:00 a.m. I was so happy not to have night sweats anymore. *Can you imagine leaving sweaty sheets behind? Can you imagine me walking out of the bedroom all wet from my hair on down? That would be even more embarrassing than the rot-gut chardonnay incident. Kind of like wetting the bed.* I don't think I would have spent the night, if I still had my night sweats. Luckily, my legs and ankles were still good enough to drive. I gathered my stuff, thanked the clan, and headed back to Glenview for an MRI.

When I got to the hospital, I took some nausea medication to help me relax for the MRI. I had a brain and neck MRI to see what was causing my strange symptoms in my extremities. I was nervous about the MRI. It was supposed to be an hour and fifteen minutes. Luckily, my nausea medicine kicked in and I almost fell asleep. I golfed and skied again. This time, I broke 100 with a 95. I almost gave myself a hole in one, but thought that was a little too much. I could have started celebrating in the machine and screwed everything up!

After the MRI, I went home to rest. I called Julie and gave her an update on my progress. She asked if I was on a special diet.

"Not really. I am trying to eat healthy. They didn't really tell me what to eat. At first, I wasn't drinking alcohol, but then they said I could. Why, what were you thinking?" I responded inquisitively, almost defensively.

"I don't know. I guess I was thinking that you should be on a special diet, because you are putting lots of poison in your body. I would think you should be supplementing the poison with something. Maybe you should see a nutritionist or take supplements. Maybe some herbs?"

My first thought was very defensive. *Leave me alone! I am doing everything they tell me to do! I am already taking chemo poison and eleven different medications!* Then, I thought about it. Julie was just trying to help her friend who was going through cancer. Everyone has their opinions and suggestions.

After my pregnant pause, I replied, "Thanks, Julie. I will ask my oncologist about it." I thought it would end with my reply, but no…

"The thing is, Vicki, most traditional doctors don't offer up non-traditional, alternative treatments that might help you feel better, especially with your strange symptoms in your arms and legs. Maybe you should see a nutritionist, acupuncturist, and chiropractor to see what suggestions they have for you."

Good intentions, good intentions, good intentions… I kept thinking, *Stop being so defensive.* After another pregnant pause, "Julie, I already have a team of doctors and am not ready to add three more to the mix." *That should end it!* Then I added, "I will see a nutritionist, if you have a suggestion."

"Great! I will email you her info." And with that, the conversation was over.

I was not in a good mood. Besides feeling tired and throbby, I had so many suggestions swirling in my head. From the suggestions from the group on my extremities, to the suggestion on the book on how I gave myself cancer, to the suggestions on alternative medicine, I was tired of hearing suggestions, even though I was asking for them. I wanted something to help my extremities. It was a long day, so I went to sleep.

July 3, 2000

I got up after a terrible night's sleep. I was aching all over. It wasn't just my extremities. It was all over. After barely any sleep, I was exhausted. I got on the scale. I had lost another two pounds. That was good news, and even without night sweats. I kept journaling every morning, but still didn't see any patterns. Maybe I would see patterns after a few more chemo sessions.

Even though it was still a holiday weekend, I forced myself to work. It was getting harder and harder to work, especially when I didn't sleep.

I worked for about four hours and got a call from my neurologist. My MRI was back, and things looked okay. *I guess that is good news?* He bumped up my Neurontin medication to help with the pain. That night, I went to the fireworks and party at the club with my mom.

July 6, 2000

My friend, Heather Mac, took me to my third chemo. It was basically the same process as the last time, except I took a CT scan before treatment, as well as the blood test. My WBC was up, and my tumors were smaller! I was so excited! The chemo was working! *Maybe I will be done in six months?!*

I introduced Heather Mac to Daniela, and the IV drip commenced. I fell asleep a few times, but was still in good spirits. We talked on and off in between my snoozing. Heather and Heather Mac were both cute, blonde friends of mine since we were about four years old. Heather Mac also had four kids, and was telling me all about them. We caught up on old high school friends. She was another close friend from preschool who was good at sports—swimming, basketball, softball, volleyball, etc. I also lived with Heather Mac for a year after college.

Dr. Kim stopped by to discuss my current situation. She asked Heather Mac to leave the room. I asked her to stay. I didn't see what the issue was whether she stayed or not. I didn't think it mattered. Dr. Kim, again, asked Heather Mac to leave the room, which she did.

This was making me nervous. Why can't she talk in front of Heather Mac? Shouldn't I be the one who decides who can listen in? Besides, my chemo brain is setting in. It is good for me to have someone there.

"Is there some reason you didn't want Heather in the room?" I asked.

"Yes. She isn't family," she curtly replied.

"That's okay. I wanted her to stay, even if she isn't family."

"I think it is better to have family members included. Don't worry. I am just here to tell you that you are on a good track. Your tumors are shrinking. Your blood work looks better. Your MRI looks good. Your CT scan looks better," she went on.

"Believe me, I'm happy about all of that, but my arms and legs still throb a lot, and I can't sleep. I am so tired all of the time. I don't think I should drive after about three in the afternoon."

"Then don't drive after 3:00," she said flippantly.

I definitely don't need this! She suggested physical therapy and wrote me a prescription. I didn't get through my list of questions for the day. I shut down.

Heather Mac came back in. "Is it safe to come back?" she asked.

"Come on in," I beamed.

"She was nice," Heather said sarcastically, rolling her eyes.

"My thoughts exactly," I confirmed.

I could switch doctors, but she was supposed to be one of the best. Obviously, her bedside manners left a lot to be desired. Daniela was a sweetheart and was the one I saw the most. I could deal with Dr. Kim from time to time, if she was making me better. That was the most important thing.

Heather Mac dropped me off back at Mom's. I told Mom about the day. She asked me a lot of questions about Dr. Kim's visit. Did you ask her this and did you ask her that? I got frustrated and went to bed early. I went to bed early to just lie there in bed...awake. I realized I had another 500 mg of steroids today. No wonder.

July 8, 2000

I had a REALLY good night's sleep. Hooray! I didn't know why. I was very thankful for the rest.

Julie took me downtown to get mail and grab clothes and go back to Mom's. I stayed at Mom's house more and more. Actually, I had moved in. Between the doctors' visits, treatments, physical therapy, the club, friends' dinners, etc., it was pretty convenient. And then there was the question of whether I could drive or not. I never knew if my ankles and legs were good enough to drive. Luckily, Julie never quizzed me on our previous discussion. I was in a good mood and didn't want to spoil it. It was very nice of her to drive me, and I was thankful.

In the afternoon, I went with my mom's friends, Nancy and Diane, to the Cancer Wellness Center for yoga. I had never done yoga before but thought this was a good way to do it. The ladies were excited too. We entered the gym with about ten other ladies of all shapes, sizes, and ages. No men. I was glad. About half of the women were wearing hats or bandanas to hide their bald heads. Everyone was wearing sweats of some sort. Leisure velour outfits *(in July?)*, college sweats, athletic sweats, tights and bodysuits, and T-shirts and shorts. I went with the T-shirt-and-short combo, no head piece. Nancy and Diane did the same.

We grabbed a mat and sat down in the back row. Then, the instructor made us all go in a circle. Bummer. I liked the back row. The yoga proceeded with a lot of breathing and some poses. I know it was supposed to be a beginner cancer patient yoga, but it was so easy anyone could do it. I guess that was the point. A child's pose was the hardest thing we had to do. I didn't learn much, but I was relaxed and could cross yoga off my list of things to try.

When I got back to Mom's house, she was not in a good mood. I usually avoided her in these moods, but there was no avoiding the wrath of Barbara when you were the target of her wrath.

"Would you take your crap upstairs? It is messing up the house," she snapped at me.

"What crap?" I asked.

"Your computer, your notebooks, and your journal are lying around all over the house."

"They are not all over the house. They are on the kitchen table. I will bring them upstairs, if that will make you happy," I snapped back.

"Yes. It would."

It is her way or the highway. I went upstairs and hid in my room until dinner to avoid further wrath. I felt like I was back in high school.

July 10, 2000

I got up, worked a few hours, and went to physical therapy.

Kirby came to town today! I was so excited to see her! She always cheered me up, just hearing her sweet voice. She was seven and very fun to be with. Kristen put her on a plane from California, and we picked her up at the gate. She came running down the jet way with her nametag and backpack on. Her blonde hair was in a ponytail. "Grandy! Aunt Vicki!" she screamed as she gave us hugs. *Now this is what I need!*

In her excited voice, Kirby babbled the whole way home in the car. She wanted to do everything, see everything, play with everything, watch everything. Exhausting! Kirby ran around the house to see her room and her toys that Mom kept there. She wanted us to play with her toys too. Aunt Vicki was at Kirby's beck and call, and Grandy joined in for a while. Soon we were watching *Singing in the Rain*, a classic, and it was time to rest.

At night, I think we were all tired. Mom got cranky. Kirby got cranky. Vicki got cranky. Between work, cranky Mom, cranky niece, and throbbing legs, I was done.

July 11, 2000

I got up and took a shower. I wasn't doing that as often these days. It took a lot of energy out of me, *so why do it, if I don't need to?* I needed to this morning. It had been a while. Unfortunately, the day had come. My hair was starting to come out as I washed it. Little clumps of hair were in my hands, and in the tub. *What a downer.* Okay, so it took three chemos to start happening. I was glad I had my wig ready to go. I didn't need it yet though.

I went downstairs and had breakfast with Mom and Kirby, which made me forget all about my hair. I went on a walk with Kirby to see some frogs nearby (Kirby was obsessed), played hopscotch (not very well), and practiced for our "show" that was to be performed for Grandy (actually very cute).

I took a nap before the big show. I needed my beauty rest to be at my best for the big show. After dinner, we had Grandy sit in a chair, and we created a little stage in front of her. Kirby was in charge of the show. She choreographed it and everything. Since we saw *Singing in the Rain* the night before, that became our show. Our costumes were raincoats and umbrellas. We used the VCR to play the song and did a little dance while twirling our umbrellas in unison. She told me what to do and I did it. I was a very good learner—*quite coachable.*

The big show lasted about a minute—definitely not more than two. At the end, we took a bow and received a standing ovation. The whole scene was so darn cute. I couldn't stop smiling and cracking up.

That night I went to bed feeling content. Even as I thought about losing my hair, I smiled. *Who cares about your hair when you have Kirby around to make you smile?*

July 14, 2000

I woke up and journaled. I had lost another pound. I thought about my extremities. I wasn't sure if physical therapy was helping or hurting me, but I did it anyway. When I woke up in the morning, my legs were pretty good and declined during the day. That pattern I noticed early on. It helped to take naps in the afternoon before going out at night. At night my legs would get so bad, I had problems getting up the stairs.

My face and neck were very swollen. I didn't look like myself in the mirror. My hair was thinning. I looked tired. Makeup didn't help. Neither did looking in the mirror. I decided to stop looking in the mirror. It didn't help anything, and it put me in a bad mood to start the day.

When I went downstairs to see Kirby and Grandy for breakfast, my mood immediately changed. I grabbed the box of Raisin Bran and poured a bowl. My tastes had changed, and my favorite things to eat were Raisin Bran, chicken, and broccoli. Most other food tasted funny to me. Kirby had her Cheerios, and Grandy had half a bagel. We were all in a good mood. Life was good.

Kristen called and we all talked to her. The human library researched my situation and thought maybe I had a paraneoplastic syndrome. A paraneoplastic syndrome is when your body creates antibodies to attack the cancer, but instead of attacking the cancer, it attacks normal cells in your nervous system. We had kind of an "ah-ha" moment. I read the information and website that my sister sent. As I read, it made sense to me. I ended up writing an email to a man who was the grand pooh-bah of paraneoplastic syndromes at Sloan Kettering, Dr. Posner. I told him all about my situation and asked him for advice. I was determined to solve my situation. Thanks to Kristen, I had hopes of doing just that.

After my internet work, I did a little work for the start-up. I was still feeling guilty about not putting too much effort into work. It was a start-up, and I should have been putting in twelve-hour days to help get it off the ground. However, I only had a few more days left with Kirby, so I did a minimal amount of work to get by and changed my focus to Kirby.

We went to the pool at the club. I slopped on a bunch of sunscreen on both of us--probably a lot more than was needed. She loved the pool and knew a number of the kids there. She was a very good swimmer, so I didn't need to worry too much about watching her every move. I joined in on the fun in the pool. The pool felt relaxing and soothing to my throbbing limbs. I made a mental note to go to the pool more often.

When Kirby was no longer entertained by the pool, we grabbed a golf cart and rode out to one of the ponds at the club. Kirby sat on my lap and steered while we drove. It was a riot. We took some bread and fed the ducks. By this time, my ankles were starting to fail for the day. Kirby was chasing the ducks, and I felt like I was one of them. My duck walk was back. I started quacking and flapping my wings. Kirby did the same. Kirby and I entertained each other for a few minutes, until I noticed some golfers watching us. This made us burst out laughing. We ran back to the cart and drove away.

Once home, I took a nap to help prepare for dinner at the Valley Lodge. The Valley Lodge and the club were my most frequented places to eat, especially when living at Mom's. It was a block away from her house. The Valley Lodge was like our *Cheers*. It was one of those places where you always knew someone there. Mom and I frequented there so much that we knew the bartender, owner, and staff very well.

The three of us ate ribs, one of their specialties. I guess the cuisine was American. Greeks owned the joint, and they had Greek items on the menu, but the ribs, filet sliders, salads, and hamburgers were fantastic. Yum. It wasn't chicken and broccoli. *I guess ribs and broccoli are on my list too.*

What a wonderful day I had. Very fulfilling! I went to bed with a smile on my face, thinking about the ducks, the pool, and Kirby.

July 17, 2000

Today was our last day with Kirby. *Boo hoo.* We ate our cereal and talked about what Kirby wanted to do before we headed to the airport. Wiffle ball and ice cream were at the top of the list. Okay, we can do that!

My ankles were in prime form for wiffle ball that morning. I wasn't going to run a marathon or anything, but I felt like I could handle wiffle ball with a seven-year-old. The three of us went outside to play in the cul-de-sac. Soon a few other kids and their parents came out to play. We were also joined by a dog. About twenty minutes into the game, we lost Kirby to the dog. So much for wiffle ball.

We stopped by Baskin Robbins on the way to the airport. Kirby got her wish once again. Mom and I ordered pralines and cream, while Kirby ordered chocolate chip cookie dough. Kirby's wish was our command. As an only child, she got spoiled, but it didn't seem to affect her. I probably spoiled her more than Grandy. I had so much joy just being with Kirby that I did almost anything she wanted. Okay, I wanted ice cream, too. After we dropped Kirby off at the airport, Mom turned to me and became solemn.

"You are really going to miss her, aren't you?"

I thought about it and gave her an honest answer. "Yes, I am. I wish they lived here. Kirby makes me so happy and makes me forget about what's going on with me. Kristen is my best friend, and I wish she was here while I go through this. She is supportive from afar, but it would be better if she were here."

"You are so good with Kirby. Does it make you want kids of your own?" she asked.

"Of course it does. You know I love kids. I have always wanted kids of my own."

"You know, Dr. Kim said that you might not be able to have kids," she reminded me.

"Yes, I know. She also said that plenty of people have had kids after ABVD. Let's cross that bridge when it comes. I am still looking for Mr. Right. I could always adopt or get a sperm donor or a dog or something, I suppose."

"Did you just say, *or a dog?*"

"Yes. I mean no. I am not comparing having a child to getting a dog, but I have been thinking about both."

"Well, either way, I am not going to be your babysitter or dog sitter," she exclaimed.

I thought this was so bizarre. *Why wouldn't she want to babysit her grandchild?* She just did with Kirby. Doesn't she want another grandchild? In addition, *why wouldn't she want to take care of my dog when I went out of town?* Not as surprising, but *really?* Maybe something was going on with her. Maybe she was menopausal or something? I wasn't in the mood to find out. I let it go. We drove the rest of the way home in silence.

July 20, 2000

Julie took me to my fourth chemo appointment. The process was the same. I went to the hospital at 8:30 a.m. to have my labs taken and was brought into my chemo room. We were waiting for Daniela, but surprisingly, Dr. Kim walked in on Julie and me.

"Hi, Dr. Kim!" Julie cheerfully announced.

"Hi, Julie. What are *you* doing here?" Dr. Kim inquired with her typical charm.

"Julie is my friend," I jumped in.

"Oh, okay. I wasn't sure if she was here in another capacity," she responded. Then she continued, "Well, your labs came back, and it looks like you may need some Neupogen for your next chemo."

"Okay. So, I can have my chemo today?" I asked, as I cringed.

"Yes. I will send in Daniela."

"Phew. I have another question. Do you think I am experiencing a paraneoplastic syndrome? I read about it online."

She kind of sneered. "Ah, I don't think so. I will pass it by Dr. Randall though."

Then, she left the room. Julie and I looked at each other and giggled.

"Wow. She was pleasant," Julie said sarcastically.

"She has a wonderful bedside manner," I replied, continuing the sarcasm. "Honestly, I don't get her. She acts like I am complaining about nothing. This is cancer. I have real symptoms. I am not sure if she is taking me seriously. I am not making this shit up. During the last chemo she kicked Heather Mac out for not being family. Apparently, you are okay to be here."

"I think she likes me, and I have dealt with a lot of cancer patients. Maybe she thinks I understand what's going on more than other people. She is a very good doctor though. Everyone says so."

"I just want this to be over! I am tired of dealing with her."

And then Daniela came in to commence the poisoning.

July 21, 2000

I had been preparing for my trip to Vancouver ever since Kirby left. The start-up management team was meeting to review strategy, forecasts, product updates, and staffing. I finished up my spreadsheets and presentation slides. This was my first in-person meeting since the diagnosis, and I wanted to be prepared. I spent most of the day packing and preparing for the meeting. I felt pretty good about it, even though I hadn't spent as much time with work as I should have.

I met the marathon runner, Hodgkin's survivor, Jeff, for lunch. I had a list of questions prepared for lunch. With my journal in tow, I walked into the restaurant looking like I was going to a business meeting, except that I was wearing shorts and a T-shirt, so maybe not. Jeff was already there, looking like he was there for a business meeting. He was a nice-looking man—blond, athletic, tan.

"It is so great to finally meet you in person, Jeff!" I began, sticking out my hand.

"Yes. I am glad this worked out," he responded with a smile, shaking my hand. There is something about a decent handshake with someone who looks you in the eye and smiles. I liked him immediately. Jeff seemed personable. We sat at a nice table in the corner. We talked a bit, ordered, and got down to business—my questions. I opened up my journal.

"I hope you don't mind. I have a list of questions for you. I am so glad that I finally get to spend some time with someone who has gone through what I am going through. I feel like everyone has other kinds of cancers with other kinds of treatments. Have you met other Hodgkin's survivors?" I asked.

"No. Not at first. I felt just like you. I couldn't find anyone. I also went to the Leukemia and Lymphoma Society for help. That's another great resource. That is partly why I volunteered at the

Cancer Wellness Center. I wanted to help other people like us. I also joined the Leukemia and Lymphoma Team in Training, while I was training for the marathon."

"It is so awesome that you ran a marathon after your treatment! I can't imagine it!"

"Well, I was a runner before, so it was a little easier for me. Although, when I finished chemo, I could barely walk."

"What? You went from not being able to walk to running a marathon?" I was shocked.

"You know, they call Hodgkin's the "cotton candy cancer" because it is highly curable. People think it is easy. The treatment is quite the opposite. How are you feeling now?"

"Tired. And I have those problems with my extremities that I told you about."

"Are you nauseous?"

"Not really. I'm not very hungry."

"Well, that's probably going to change. I was sick as a dog. I was extremely exhausted and weak. I had bad chemo brain too."

"Oh! I think I have started getting chemo brain. My memory is fuzzy and forgetful. I have to write down everything. Hence, the journal…"

"I noticed that. Keeping a journal is a good idea. I wish I had done it."

Lunch lasted an hour and a half. Jeff was incredible. I was thankful to have him as a resource. I had three pages of notes from our lunch. I hoped I didn't get him in trouble with work. I tried to buy, but he wouldn't let me; so we split it. We hugged and parted ways. What a nice guy. *Why are all the nice guys taken?*

I felt conflicted about lunch. Obviously, I was not excited about the thought of being sick as a dog. I supposed if that's the price you have to pay to be cancer-free, then pay it. If Jeff could do it, I could do it. But then again, Jeff was a marathon runner, and I was not about to do that. The farthest I had run was eight miles.

On the bright side, I had a new friend and/or resource. Jeff told me I could call him any time. It seemed a lot easier to call him with a simple question or thought than waiting for a visit with Dr. Kim. He was warm and friendly too.

July 23–29, 2000

I flew to Vancouver for my meeting with the start-up. I felt prepared for the meeting but unsure about my health. It was a very long flight, and I wasn't sure how my extremities would handle it. Walking through the airport was a nightmare. My legs were very numb and weak. I had to rest a few times before getting to my gate at O'Hare. Luckily, I got an upgrade to first class due to my many miles flown with the corporation. My legs were throbbing the whole flight. I watched a few movies and slept.

The week consisted of a blur of internal and external meetings; that is, internal management and sales team meetings, and external client and partner meetings. I had a pretty aggressive schedule with a plan to rest between meetings and at night. It was difficult managing and balancing my work and health issues, especially since my chemo brain was setting in. I definitely was not in prime form.

On the way home, I made sure I had wheelchair assistance through the airport. It was kind of fun flying through the airport in a wheelchair. My legs were much better on the flight home too.

The Vancouver meetings were declared a success in my mind but not an overwhelming success. Overall, I would give the meetings a B. I should have felt okay with that, but I was used to getting As, not Bs. I would give my health a solid D, but that was par for the course for my millennium.

July 29, 2000

I slept in after my long week in Vancouver. I needed it. I started my usual morning process at Mom's house. I met her downstairs for breakfast, which consisted of a bowl of Raisin Bran and a Diet Coke. *Strange, huh?* Mom had what she called a "cheese goody": toast with melted Swiss cheese on it. She sat and read the paper, giving me the Chicago sports highlights. She had the SCORE radio program on in the background while reading the paper. I never bothered her in the morning during her ritual, and she never bothered me during mine. Breakfast: check.

After breakfast I had my usual handful of pills and watched the *Today Show*. The SCORE was a part of her process, and the *Today Show* was a part of mine. I was banished to my room for mine, which was fine with me. Pills: check.

I watched while I wrote in my journal. I documented my health: limbs—constantly numb, tingling, throbbing, and weak; hair—slowly falling out, but no need for the wig yet; nausea—none; face and neck—swollen; chemo brain—spacey and forgetful. Journal: check.

The last step to my process was to get dressed for the day, which I skipped some days. I was typically quite casual—shorts or leggings and a shirt. I was getting tired of my clothes at my mom's house. I needed to head back downtown to retrieve some other clothes and mail soon. Dressed: check.

Once my process was complete, I went to physical therapy. I hadn't been in a week. I hadn't done my exercises either. I wasn't sure if the exercises were helping my limbs at all, but I had to try something.

Next, I went to play golf with Mom. I didn't want to play with anyone else, because I didn't know how long I would last or how I would do with my duck feet and numb limbs. The notion of wanting to solely play with my mom was kind of odd. My mom used to force me to play golf as a kid; hence, my original hatred of the sport. Since then, I learned to love the game due to having a boyfriend with a 3 handicap.

It was wonderful to be out on the course with a beautiful day in the 70s and not a cloud in the sky. I was a bit wobbly, weak, and off-balance. I didn't keep score. I just wanted to play. On the par 3 eighth hole, I hit it into the green-side sand trap. I grabbed the rake, wobbled into the trap, and proceeded to hit my shot.

"SHIT!" I yelled loudly, as I lost what little balance I had and fell backward into the trap with my arms and club flailing in the air. It was a full-on fall into the sand, losing my hat, club, sunglasses, and pride. The trap looked like what skiers would call a yard sale when they have a bad wipeout. I scrambled around the trap for my belongings and raked the trap, hoping nobody saw my wipeout. Mom was immediately horrified at my scream heard around the course, as she looked around to see who heard me. The coast was clear. *I will never forget that trap wipeout as long as I live.*

With all of the commotion, I had no idea where I hit my ball. I looked up and saw that it was right next to the pin. I actually had a par! Wow!

We finished the hole and started walking off the green when *whammo!* A golf ball from the second hole came flying at my mom and hit her in the mouth. Then, it was my mom's turn to scream. Blood was gushing from her mouth. I ran over to her with a towel to find out that she kept all of her teeth in the incident. Phew!

We jumped into the golf cart and drove to the clubhouse as fast as the little cart would allow. Luckily, we were on the eighth hole and close. The club manager ran over with a bag of ice—Mom's savior. Knowing my mom, this scene could have gone in a lot of different directions. It could have been a near-death experience, in which she wanted to sue for attempted manslaughter, or it could have been no big deal in which she wanted to be left alone. Today, she graced us with playing it on the down low. *Yes!*

We cleaned all of the blood, sweat, and sand off of ourselves in the locker room and sat on the terrace for dinner. Mom got sympathy from the club members who walked by as the news had spread about her being hit by a ball. The experience was very scary, but she was fine, and you couldn't even tell by looking at her that she had just been hit.

I wouldn't call it a successful golf outing. In fact, I had no desire to go back out and play. I will always remember the tragic eighth-hole experience every time I play the hole—it wasn't all bad though; I had a par.

July 31, 2000

After I finished my process, I went to physical therapy and headed to the airport. I had a client meeting in Mobile, Alabama. I was going to meet with a man named Doug Dip. I didn't know the client personally, so I started to envision all kinds of things. I know it is stereotyping, but I couldn't help thinking that Doug Dip looked scruffy, had a big old accent, had little to no teeth, and had dip stuck in his teeth. My imagination was running wild as I prepared for the meeting.

I wheel chaired through O'Hare to save my legs from the walk. The flight was fine. My stereotyping of Mobile, Alabama, started out to be true when I first landed at the airport. I rented a car that ended up being a souped-up Dodge Charger, just like in *The Dukes of Hazzard*. I was driving the General Lee. No kidding! Fortunately, my legs were good enough to drive. I planned the trip to get to Mobile early enough to be able to drive while my legs were still good. I checked into the hotel.

By the time I got to my room, I was exhausted. I lay down on the bed and started watching the movie *Flashdance*. My legs and arms gradually became their worst ever. They were extremely numb and throbbing. I couldn't imagine meeting with Doug Dip in the morning. My mind started taking over as I lay there in misery. I could hardly watch the movie. *What was I thinking? Why am I wheel chairing through airports trying to work? Am I crazy?* My mind went darker. *Am I going to survive this? What if I die? My dad died at fifty-eight. I could die at thirty-four.* For the first time during this illness, I actually thought I could be dying. Then, it went lighter. *If I ever get healthy again, I am going to do whatever it takes to stay healthy the rest of my life. I choose not to die from cancer!*

I picked up the phone and called my sis, Kris. No answer. I called Bryan. He was at the airport on a work trip and answered immediately in his usual upbeat voice, "What's up, Vick?"

"I'm not doing too well, Bryan," I responded weakly.

"Aw, what's wrong?"

"I am in Mobile, Alabama, for a meeting tomorrow, and I don't feel so good. I am lying in bed at the hotel and am extremely exhausted and throbbing all over," I cried. "I can't stand this anymore!" I launched into a full-on sob.

After a long pause, he said, "Why don't you cancel the appointment? I am sure they will understand."

"I can't cancel! I have had this set for a long time. I NEED to do this!"

"Some things you need to do for your health, Vicki."

"I promise, I will cancel in the morning, if I am not better. I am sorry to bother you, but I am frustrated and need someone to talk to. You are the lucky one who answered their phone."

"It'll be okay, Vicki. You are just going through a bad time. Rest up, get a good night's sleep, and I am sure you will feel better in the morning. Next time, can someone else make the sales call? I don't think you should be running across the country like this when you are trying to recover from cancer." He had a good point. *What am I doing?*

"Good point, Bry. Thanks for listening to me. I appreciate it. Now go catch your flight."

I felt better. It helped just to talk to someone. It felt good to cry. I think I kept a lot in and needed to release it. Bryan just happened to be the target. Next time I would have to pick someone else to release on. You know. Share the pain.

After looking in the mirror, I wrote in my journal: *Don't look good, don't feel good, but I am good.*

Chapter Eight

August 2000: My Leave

> "We all have problems. But it's not what happens to us, [it's] the choices we make after."
>
> — *Elizabeth Smart*

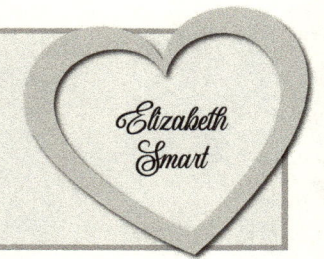

August 1, 2000

After twelve hours of sleep I was ready to go. I did a fast-track process to make sure I was on time for Doug Dip. I jumped into my car, the General Lee, and sped off to see Mr. Dip. I was pleasantly surprised to meet Doug. I was wrong. He was a tall, tan, slender man, dressed in khakis and a button-down: no accent, no dip, clean shaven, great handshake, nice smile with teeth.

Doug and I had a productive meeting, resulting in a number of follow-up action items on both of our parts. That was my goal, so I deemed the meeting successful.

We had lunch in their cafeteria while we chatted about life and sports. My stereotyping of Doug Dip couldn't have been further from the truth. He was a transplant from the northeast and an avid golfer. He told me about the Robert Trent Jones Golf Trail that runs throughout the state, which he highly recommended. A lot of the courses were already built, and they were continuing to expand across the state. I always knew golf was good for business—talking it and playing it.

After lunch, I jumped in the General Lee, like Daisy Duke, and drove back to the airport feeling content. I was in such a good mood. I couldn't believe how low I felt the day before. A twelve-hour sleep and attitude adjustment were just what I needed.

That night, back at Mom's, I told her about my trip. It was probably a mistake to tell her about the scene at the hotel. She told me how ridiculous it was for me to keep working. I always took these discussions with Mom with a grain of salt.

August 2, 2000

After completing my process, I worked for a few hours, went to physical therapy, swam some laps at the pool, and went to the Cancer Wellness Center. I had a session on "healing touch." I signed up for this free session, unsure of what it was supposed to do for me, but I was up for anything that could make me feel better.

I lay on a massage table while a young woman touched me at specific spots on my body. While breathing incense slowly and deeply, her calm voice and soft touch almost made me fall asleep. I was so relaxed, practically dozing off, until I started sneezing. I had a surprisingly loud, high-pitched sneeze. I think I scared the shit out of the clinician, who probably thought I was asleep. *Ahhchoooo!* Again and again, I sneezed. The "healing touch" was halted at once. The toucher stepped back and asked if I was okay, while handing me a tissue. "Sure," I responded, "I guess I ruined the mood."

So, I checked "healing touch" off of my list of things to try. I had tried physical therapy, swimming, medications, supplements, healing touch, and yoga. I thought healing touch would be more like a massage, but it wasn't. I still had acupuncture, chiropractor, massage, and meditation left to try. And maybe biofeedback, but I didn't know what that was.

I went back to Mom's and took a nap. Afterward, I worked a bit and filled out an application for a handicap placard for my car. Mom had been nagging me about it for a while now, and it was time I did it. I was weaker and weaker and it was about time. Unfortunately, I had no idea how long the state would take to fulfill my needs. My guess was about a month.

I was happy to see a note from the famous Dr. Posner. He thought I was doing the right things for my extremities. He thought I should have a lumbar puncture to help determine the cause of my extremity issue. He neither confirmed nor denied paraneoplastic syndrome. He invited me to Sloan Kettering to be examined by his team. I was seriously considering the invite. I followed up with an email.

August 3, 2000

It was Chemo Day once again. This time my friend Sue took me. I went early for my blood test, which was fine. No Neupogen needed. I introduced Sue to Daniela and watched a movie. The chemo process went smoothly. I stayed awake laughing with Sue as the chemo dripped through my veins. We were watching the movie *Arthur* and talking during the commercials. We reminisced about the good old days of high school and all of the trouble we got in.

As we reminisced, Sue reminded me of the Notre Dame revelation. My dad had season tickets and parking passes to Notre Dame football games. We even went to the Sugar Bowl in 1973 for the Notre Dame vs. Alabama championship game. My dad hummed the fight song around the house. One day, I explained to Sue that my dad was humming the fight song because it was game day and his school, Notre Dame, was playing. My dad stopped in his tracks and corrected me. "I didn't go to Notre Dame. I went to Wabash."

"What?! I thought you went to Notre Dame? Then why are we such big fans? Why do we go to all of the games?" I inquired.

"Tradition! Our whole family was born and raised Notre Dame football fans. Notre Dame is the best school and has the best football team in the land."

Boy, did I feel dumb. I had been telling people for years that my dad went to Notre Dame. Sue just laughed. She laughed at me back in high school and she laughed at me while poison was dripping into my veins. "Okay, very funny, Sue." I chuckled.

August 5, 2000

After my morning process, I drove Mom to the airport. I was tremendously bummed about not going on the family Idaho rafting trip. I loved rafting. I loved the wilderness. I loved fishing. I loved camping. I loved my cousins.

I was in a quiet mood. Mom, on the other hand, was not. She was babbling about all of the things on her list for me to do while she was out of town. Her/my to-do list was quite lengthy. Watering her flowers was at the top of her list. I was going to be a dead woman if her flowers died. I was also cautioned to not overwater the flowers too. It almost made me nervous taking over such a huge responsibility as watering the flowers.

My family was totally out of touch with humanity on the rafting trip. The only communication they had was a satellite phone to be used for emergencies only. I had the number of the outfitter on the to-do list, in case I had an emergency. Mom was worried about leaving me alone. I was not sure what could have happened while she was gone, but I had the number, just in case.

Mom, Kristen, Bryan, Kirby, and twenty of my cousins took a rafting trip down the Salmon River in Idaho for a week. Dr. Kim decided it was too much for me. I guess she was right. At sixty-one, Mom was the oldest and "matriarch" on the trip. Kirby just made the cut-off, as the youngest at seven. Three guides led them down the river with various-sized rafts and kayaks, camping at a different location every night. Once they stopped at a campsite, the guides set up camp, with a bar located in the middle containing booze pre-ordered by the team. They were notified that their booze order was the biggest ever ordered at the outfitter. *That's my family!*

Idaho had a huge wildfire that summer, and the trip was almost canceled. They had to pick their campsites carefully, so they didn't have to deal with embers or smoke.

When I dropped Mom off and gave her a big hug I started crying. *Why am I crying?* I wasn't sure why, but I had been feeling emotional about the littlest things. I cried at anything. I should have been happy. I had the week to myself. *What wild and crazy things can I do?* I went home and took a nap.

When I woke up, I felt extremely nauseous. I didn't throw up, but I felt like it. I suppose this was what Marathon Jeff was talking about. The nausea had begun, and I wasn't happy about it. I called Bill and canceled dinner with him. That was the last thing I felt like doing. I hung out and watched TV the rest of the day and night, falling asleep here and there.

August 6, 2000

Feeling lethargic, I started my process a little late today as I lingered in bed for longer than usual. With my breakfast partner being out of town, I wasn't in a hurry to go downstairs. I analyzed my health and documented it in my journal. "Emotional" and "nauseous" were my new additions to the list. Bummer. On the other hand, my legs were feeling pretty good.

Although it was Sunday, I did some work in the morning. It was getting harder and harder to focus as my chemo brain got worse and worse. I tried to work as much as possible every day, especially in the morning. With my brain functioning slower, it took twice as long to do anything. Two hours of work was about all I could handle.

Giving up on work on a gorgeous day, I headed to the pool for lunch and swimming—Sunday Funday. My friend Cynthia saved me a spot in our usual location by the diving board. Not only did it have the best sun, it was entertaining watching the kids go off the diving board. We had lunch with her three kids, while her husband played golf. Cynthia and I grew up as pool brats at the club. She and her family were terrific swimmers.

After lunch, I slopped on the sunscreen and read my book. I started reading books on cancer. I was picky about the cancer books I bought. I wanted to make sure they were positive, light-hearted books about survivors. There was no reason to get depressed. I was reading a funny book by Julia Sweeney from *Saturday Night Live*. The book was about her brother having cancer. I was enjoying it until I discovered her brother died. I stopped reading it and switched to my *People* magazine.

Cynthia and I were joined by more friends as the day went on. The Sunday afternoon drinks kicked off with rum stone sours flowing. The men came over to the pool after golf and eventually it turned into "Family Fun Night." Margie and Hugh's family joined us. The club had an early dinner buffet, which was perfect for us. Our group commandeered the diving area as the adults began to take over the board. The biggest splash contest was a big hit, as well as pool brats from long ago showing off their talents from long ago.

After taunting from the kids, Hugh did a double flip. *Show off!* More taunting. Cynthia did a flip. More taunting. Margie did a flip. Then others who had no business being on the diving board joined in, including me. I was a sucker under peer pressure, especially from kids. As they yelled, "Flip, flip, flip," I waddled to the end of the board and jumped as high as I could while trying to fling my body around. *Splat!* I didn't make it the whole way around and was still in a tuck. Oh well. I tried.

Another thing Aunt Vicki liked to do with the kids was be the prime target for them to push me in the water. I stood on the edge of the pool talking to Margie as a couple of the kids snuck up behind me. With one well-coordinated shove, I went flying into the pool, letting out a loud scream. This occurred every Family Fun Night, and I loved it.

I went home and crashed. *What an amazing Sunday Funday I had with some amazing friends!*

August 11, 2000

I spent the following weekend downtown at my place. I didn't feel like doing much, but I had plans and I made myself follow through on my commitments. If I was going to feel shitty, I might as well do it in the company of friends. My energy level was low, and I generally felt like crap: tired, cranky, throbbing, numb, and my new favorite, nauseous. I took nausea medicine, but it didn't help much. I made the mistake of looking in the mirror. My hair was thin. My face and neck were bloated. I wish it was the other way around—thin face and neck, and bloated hair.

I relaxed most of the day. I worked for a while and took a nap. In the afternoon, I went to the Field Museum with Cate and Julie to see Sue, the T-Rex dinosaur. It was a blast. We cruised through the Sue crowd with ease using my wheelchair to part the crowd. I felt like I should have brought a horn—*Beep beep, cancer person coming through!* We had so much fun, we decided we needed to hit up all of the museums with wheelchairs. We'd save that for another day.

After the Field Museum, we headed over to Rush and Division Streets, otherwise known as the Viagra Triangle. We had a drink at Gibson's and then at Hugo's Frog Bar next door. Both places had a piano player for entertainment. I always enjoyed piano bars.

I looked around for Bill. He liked to hang out there. None of my friends had met Bill. As I thought about it, I can't believe I met Bill in the Viagra Triangle of all places. Or maybe I can. I chuckled as I thought about it.

August 12, 2000

I had another lazy morning in bed after my big day out. My morning process took about two hours. I didn't care though. I had to be ready to go by 3:00 p.m. for pregaming at Butch's before the Bears preseason game. Kurt and I both had four season tickets to the Chicago Bears games. We either tailgated in the parking lot or went to Butch McGuire's and took a bus to the game. Today was a Butch's day. I put on my uniform, which consisted of my Gary Fencik jersey from the '85 Bears team, shorts, Bears shoes, Bears beads, Bears earrings, and Bears cap to hide my thin hair. I walked down the street and took a cab to the bar.

Butch's was a festive, historic Irish bar in the Viagra Triangle. It was loaded with Bears fans of all ages, shapes, and sizes wearing blue and orange. I scanned the room, checking out the crowd for my friends, but also for possible single men. Considering the high volume of thirty-something male football fans in attendance, I was in the right place. I know I gave up the "man" goal for "my millennium," but it was a habit. I couldn't help myself from checking out the crowd. My friends had started gathering at a table in the front. They were waving me over, so my man scan didn't last very long.

We had a table for eight in the front of the bar next to the open windows—best table in the house. I had a prime seat for the man scan as they were coming and going to and from the bar as well as the bonus sidewalk. Heather, Kurt, Cate, Julie, and a few of Kurt's buddies were there. It was fun sitting next to the window as people walked by high-fiving and yelling, "Go Bears!" We were getting pumped up for the game.

When it was time to go to the game we jumped in the party bus stocked with a keg of beer. Butch's wasn't far from the stadium, but in football traffic, it took about forty minutes to get there. Forty minutes to drink a keg of beer—and it was gone!

The guys sat in Kurt's seats near the fifty-yard line, and the girls sat in my end-zone seats. It was just a preseason game, so it wasn't critical to actually watch the game. The Bears haven't been very good since the '85 Super Bowl Championship team. We have been rebuilding ever since. Dick Jauron was our coach, and he was a nice guy and all, but we didn't win many games. We were hoping to turn that around with our new linebacker, Brian Urlacher. We were excited to see Urlacher, but that's about it. We were playing the Browns and won, but that's not saying much; the Browns were traditionally even worse than the Bears.

I ended up going home at halftime, so I watched the end of the game at home in bed. I hit a wall in the second quarter and quit while I was ahead for the day. Julie wouldn't let me go home alone, so she took a cab with me. Thank God she did, because I was really having problems walking to find one. I was extremely weak and held on to her arm while she led me to the cab line. I almost fell a few times, taking her down with me. Eventually, we made it to the cab, and I fell asleep quickly, while making the trek back to Lincoln Park. Julie paid for the cab and woke me up when we pulled up to my place. She wasn't satisfied until she got me up the stairs and into bed, with the Bears game on, of course.

All in all a great day and a Bears win!

August 13, 2000

I had another lazy morning in bed. I put on the TV as I was going through my process and writing in my journal. On weekdays, I watched the *Today Show*, and on weekends I watched *Meet the Press*. They were my regular shows that were on in the background while I worked my way through my process. I saw a General Electric commercial talking about their CT scan machines, and my mind started wandering. I certainly had my share of CT scans and MRIs. I felt like maybe that is something I could do—sell CT scan and MRI machines. With my engineering, sales, and scanning experience, I would be good at that. I could talk from the patient's point of view and was able to talk techie. I made a note in my journal.

I packed up some clothes and headed up north to Glenview. Mom had just gotten home from her trip and couldn't wait to tell me all about it at dinner. But first, I had a lunch to go to. It's kind of funny. The only things I had to do today were lunch and dinner, and I had zero appetite. I was already strategizing—chicken soup for lunch, and chicken and broccoli for dinner.

It was Sunday Funday once again. However, this time I had lunch at the club with my fellow cancer patients and yoga stars, Diane and Nancy (Mom's friends). Again, it was one of those amazing days in August with a high of eighty degrees and not a cloud in the sky. We ate on the terrace next to the eighteenth green of the golf course. My sun paranoia settled in and I slopped on some sunscreen. They both made fun of me for slopping on the sunscreen. "Vicki, you don't need that much sunscreen," Nancy said.

"Well, you can never be too careful. They told me to watch out. The chemo makes you burn very easily." Secretly, I thought of my dad dying of melanoma.

Diane chimed in, "Nothing could get through that much sunscreen. You look like a ghost. They just want you to be careful. You don't have to overboard. By the way, how is your chemo going? How are you feeling?"

"I have my sixth one this week. I feel okay. My arms and legs still bother me. I am pretty tired most of the time. My hair started falling out. I am nauseous all of the time now. Have you taken anything special that works for nausea?" I was always looking for answers.

Nancy replied, "Get that wig ready! When your hair starts to get fuzzy, you should shave it off and start wearing your wig. That should be any time now. Unfortunately, I never found anything that works for nausea. Sorry. Have you, Diane?"

"No. I don't have much nausea."

"I have been taking Marinol, which is supposed to have some form of marijuana in it. It doesn't seem to do anything for me. Have either of you taken that?" I asked.

"I tried it. I agree. I don't think it helps, so I stopped taking it," Nancy affirmed.

I think she has tried everything. She had breast cancer twice.

Diane added, "Never tried it. Hey, Nancy, didn't you get a scan this week?"

"Yes! I am all good. Thank God!" Nancy announced.

"Wow! Awesome! What wonderful news!" I cheered.

"You've been keeping this from us, Nancy! I am so happy for you!"

"I don't know. I don't want to get too excited. It has already come back once." Nancy played it on the down low. I understood. I am not sure I would be doing backflips if I had already had a recurrence.

I am glad we had something to celebrate. It was not just a beautiful Sunday Funday, but it was encouraging to see a fellow cancer survivor achieve a significant goal. *Can I call myself a survivor yet?* It was like we were a team fighting our biggest common rival and enemy, cancer. All for one and one for all.

After our lunch celebration, I went to Mom's and took a nap. The great rafting trip stories would have to wait until dinner. Wow! I ended up sleeping for three hours! I am not sure if it was the busy weekend, or maybe just the fact that I had a ton of poison in my body killing these bad boys in my chest. It was probably both.

By the time I came downstairs, Mom was already cooking dinner. Guess what! It was chicken and broccoli! She had me pegged. I was sure she was going to get sick of making chicken and broccoli. She always made a little something extra, so she didn't get too sick of eating chicken and broccoli.

I played with my food as Mom told me the story of her trip. I had a bite every once in a while, then picked and stirred.

"We all missed you and wished you were there. It was an once-in-a-lifetime experience that we should do again—with you next time. Maybe it was a twice-in-a-lifetime experience. Everything was first class. They made roughing it not so rough. It took us a whole day to get there. We flew into Boise, puddle-jumped to the area, and then a bussed to the drop-in location. The Salmon River was mostly class two and three rapids. I usually stayed in a raft we called Cleopatra's Barge. It was the biggest raft that carried all of our belongings and up to ten people.

"Every once in a while I took a single kayak. One time I was paddling in a kayak down some tough rapids and I went flying out of the kayak and down the rapids. I almost died! I could have died! I have never been so scared in my life! Everyone was yelling at me, but I couldn't get to the side. One of the guides had to come save me."

"Oh my gosh, Mom! Are you all right?"

"Yes. I am perfectly fine, but I thought I was going to die!" She was shaking as she was talking, so it obviously really scared her. She calmed down and finished telling me about the trip.

After dinner, I headed to the couch. Mom and I had our usual spots in the living room. She had the love seat and I had the couch. I kept a plastic wastebasket by my couch just in case I needed it for the chicken and broccoli.

We watched *60 Minutes*, one of my mom's favorites. Then, we watched *Sex and the City*, one of my favorites. I had been telling my mom about the show for a few years and this was her first time watching it.

Boy, was that a mistake! The one episode my mom happened to see involved Samantha having a vivid, illicit lesbian relationship with lots of sex.

"What kind of garbage do you watch, Vicki?! This is disgusting!" she burst out. "I can't believe you like this trash!"

"I swear, Mom. This is the worst it has been! I have never seen an episode like this! Let's watch something else!"

And just like that, we put on AMC.

August 14, 2000

After my morning process, Mom and I went to the hospital to see Dr. Randall about the possibility of me having a paraneoplastic syndrome. Dr. Kim had spoken to him about it.

"I thought about that as a possibility, but I don't think so. We can rule it out with a lumbar puncture. We can do it now, if you would like?"

I got excited. "Sure! Let's do it!"

My mom was not so sure, "Hang on. What's a lumbar puncture?"

"I need to take some fluid out of your spinal column. It is also referred to as a spinal tap."

"Does it hurt?" she asked.

"We will make sure she doesn't feel a lot of pain."

"Okay, let's do it," Mom said, unassured.

The lumbar puncture would have been just fine if the doctor got it right the first time he punctured me. However, it wasn't so straightforward. Apparently, it is not so simple to puncture the spinal column with the needle. I guess you have to hit it just right. It took four times to get it right. Each time, I squeezed my mom's hand for dear life. Her hand was turning purple. I had sweat dripping down my back and off my nose. I became light-headed. *Why am I putting myself through this?* I had to know what was afflicting my extremities so badly. I wanted it to stop. I would do anything to help my extremities.

We were told we would have the results in forty-eight hours.

August 17, 2000

Chemo Day! It was my friend Robin's turn to take me to chemo. Robin and I attended *every* year in school together, including college at Southern Methodist University. We even, unintentionally, ended up on the same freshman floor together. *Is that fate, coincidence, or what?*

I gave Robin a heads up. "I really appreciate you taking me to chemo, but, FYI, I will probably fall asleep and cry. I can't help it."

"No problem, Vick. I am just going to sit here and watch TV."

My blood levels were fine. Chemo went relatively smoothly. It seemed like I had a new discovery every chemo session. This chemo session, I had this metallic taste in my mouth the whole time. It was like I tasted the poison while it was going into my body. It was such a strange sensation.

I fell asleep and woke up to Dr. Randall. "Hi, Vicki."

"Hi," I said groggily. "What's up?"

"I have your results from the lumbar puncture. We found no antibodies in the fluid that would potentially attack your nervous system."

I began to cry and fell back to sleep. *I guess I don't have a paraneoplastic syndrome?*

Robin had the luck of being the one to try to cheer me up after the news. Between the effect of the poison and results of the lumbar puncture, I was a mess. She did the best she could. Soon, Robin dropped me at Mom's house and I went back to sleep.

August 19, 2000

On Mom's quest to make the millennium as fun as possible for me, she planned a staycation downtown. We packed up the car in the morning and headed down to The Drake hotel. Luckily, our room was ready, and we put our stuff in the room. We changed our clothes and headed to the Oak Street Beachstro for the Air and Water Show. The Drake was the perfect location for the Air and Water Show, because it was just across Lake Shore Drive from the beach. The Oak Street Beachstro was a new beach-themed restaurant on Oak Street Beach, a prime location for the show. The weather was a high of eighty-five degrees and sunny—ideal for the show! I slopped on some sunscreen, including some spray sunscreen that Robin had given me for my slightly balding head. Apparently, her dad wore it golfing.

The radio station 1000 AM was broadcasting the show nearby—also, ideal for the show. We were kept abreast of everything that was going on in the show, backstories and all. I had zero appetite but managed to enjoy the food and drinks. Actually, after my second champagne I got hungry. *Bonus!* The show ended with the Blue Angels flying through the buildings of the city. *Very cool.* I handled the walk to and fro the show with no problems, *also ideal.* We were having an ideal day. We took a nap at The Drake and went to the Pump Room for dinner to cap off our ideal day.

This time, there were no celebrities at the Pump Room, but there was a lounge singer to entertain us during dinner. To end our ideal day, we went back to The Drake to the Coq Dor for more lounge singing and a nightcap. The piano player, Craig, was incredible! And adorable! And about my age! We met Craig during a break. We bought him a drink and he sat with us. Apparently, he played football at Notre Dame. Okay, adorable *and* played football at Notre Dame! Now, he had my attention.

"Wow, I can't believe you played football at Notre Dame! We are huge Notre Dame fans!" I exclaimed.

"Yeah, it was amazing! I was in the ROTC program."

"What position did you play?" I asked him.

"Running back," he responded.

"That's awesome!"

"Well, yes, but I only got one play in four years and I fumbled the ball."

I couldn't help giggling. I felt bad, but I couldn't help it. I laughed. "I'm sorry for laughing." And then I quickly changed the subject.

We listened to Craig a while longer and went up to bed. I was exhausted, but what a wonderful day!

August 21, 2000

After my morning process, I jumped in the car and headed for cheeseland. I had a meeting with a small company in Milwaukee. I scheduled it for the late morning, so I would be at my best physically and mentally. Or so I thought.

I was on I-94 up around the Wisconsin border listening to the radio when my chemo brain set in. Suddenly, I had no idea where I was or where I was going or why. I pulled off the road at Racine. Once I was safely off the road, I sat and pondered. *Where am I going? Why am I going to Wisconsin?* I looked down at my passenger seat and saw my computer bag and remembered my sales call. *Oh wow! Is this really happening? Am I losing it? Am I getting dementia?* I pulled back on the road, drove to Milwaukee, and handled my sales call quite well, despite having dementia.

August 25, 2000

I slept in. I went down for breakfast around ten in the morning. Mom was already finished with the morning paper and bustling around the house listening to her buddies on the SCORE radio program. It was gameday for the Bears, so there was a lot of football talk. I ate my Raisin Bran as she walked in.

"I think today is the day," she said.

"Today is the day for what?" I inquired.

"Today is the day you are going to quit your job."

I think she was bracing for an argument from me. I had been thinking about it constantly, especially since my recent dementia experience. I was not doing my health situation any good by stressing out over my job. And, I was not doing the start-up any good by doing a half-assed job at sales. They needed someone who was not burdened with fighting cancer, chemo, doctors' appointments, chemo brain, nausea, and fatigue. They needed someone who could focus.

"I think you are right, Mom. I am going to call Marc today."

Shocked, Mom exploded, "That's terrific! You will be able to go to Italy with a clear head and not think about anything else, but having a fabulous time!"

The Italy trip had nothing to do with it, but I guess she was right. I think I had made the decision weeks ago, but it felt good to finalize the decision, and it felt even better to actually call Marc and do it. I called him right after breakfast.

"Hi, Marc, how are you?"

"Hey, Vicki. The bigger question is, how are *you?*"

"Doing okay. Same old, same old, nausea, fatigue, brain fog. I am calling to ask you if I can take a leave of absence for the rest of my chemo treatments. I feel like I am not doing myself or the company any good by working like this. You deserve better than that."

"Well, I don't know about that, but I was wondering the same thing. It is probably better to have you focus completely on getting well. I am surprised we haven't talked about this sooner. You shouldn't have to worry about work. I was thinking that you should keep the car, computer, phone, and company shares, and hopefully you come back when you are feeling better and ready to go."

"That sounds great. I feel really bad about this, but I think it is the right thing to do for all of us."

We discussed an exit plan with transferring accounts, knowledge, and information, but besides that, I was done. It felt liberating.

That afternoon, we packed up the car and went to Soldier Field to tailgate with Heather and Kurt before the Bears game. I had my new handicap placard, so we could park right next to the stadium. That was one bonus to having cancer that I hadn't thought of. I felt bad taking up a handicap spot, but I deserved it for everything I was going through. The four of us grilled steaks and veggies for dinner before the game. It was quite tasty. We toasted to my quitting the start-up. We were celebrating.

We lost to the Tennessee Titans. It was still preseason, so it didn't really matter, but I didn't like to lose. We left early again. I made it until the fourth quarter this time. That's progress.

August 31, 2000

Another high school friend, Karen, took me to chemo. They sent me into radiology for a quick x-ray and the lab for my bloodwork. My labs were fine, and the process commenced after a discussion with Daniela. I had accumulated a long list of questions in my journal to go over. I wasn't sure if my questions were for Daniela or Dr. Kim, so I started with Daniela.

"I feel like I am bruising more easily now. Is that due to the chemo?" I asked.

"Yes. That is normal," Daniela responded.

"My nausea seems to be getting worse. Is that normal?"

"Yes. Your nausea should increase as you have more and more chemo."

"I haven't gotten my period since I started taking chemo. Is that normal?"

"Yes."

"I think my skin and eyes are really dry. Is that from chemo?"

"Probably. I would use eye drops and lotion."

"I feel like my vision is declining. Could that be from the chemo?"

"Maybe. I think you should see your eye doctor. Maybe drops would help."

And so on…

It was a typical chemo: in and out of sleep, crying, TV, and catching up with Karen. Dr. Kim came in to visit with me at the end. She asked Karen to leave while she gave me my x-ray results. Again, I told her that Karen could stay, but she insisted that Karen leave. Apparently, according to the x-ray, there was no change in the tumors. I was pretty bummed. She tried to say a few words of comfort, but Dr. Kim was not very comforting. She was pretty straightforward, which was good and bad. She certainly didn't sugarcoat anything. I guess I always knew where I stood with her, but that didn't make me feel any better.

After I was given the news, Karen drove me home. It seemed like Karen was okay with the experience, because she offered to take me again. I guess I wasn't the worst company or too boring to hang out with for six hours doing nothing.

Chapter Nine
September 2000: My Wig

> "Keep your face always toward the sunshine, and shadows will fall behind you."
>
> — Walt Whitman

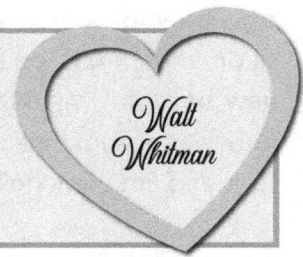

September 1-2, 2000

After successfully quitting my job, transferring knowledge, and completing my seventh chemo, I was ready to go to Italy with my mom. *Let the adventure begin!*

I had been packing for a week in preparation for the big trip. I loaded up with hats, sunscreen, medication, my wig, walking shoes, bathing suits, and clothes. I had been to Italy before, but I was touring, and this was going to be completely different. I was going to relax and enjoy myself. I was going to be pampered. I was really looking forward to it. Mom's efforts to make my cancer journey bearable and fun were about to really begin with Italy. *And, who knows? Maybe I am about to meet my perfect man from far, far away.*

I was also excited to wear my new wig. I had been wearing various baseball caps to hide my hair loss. Now, it was time to bring out the big guns. A few days before we left for Italy, I went to my hairdresser who cut my hair (fuzz) and shaved my head in the back room of the salon. It was so thoughtful of her to take me into the back, so we could be discreet during the buzz cut. I didn't want everyone in the salon to see me get a fuzz buzz. It is a very personal experience, especially for a woman. It actually wasn't so bad. I walked into the salon with "fuzz" on my head and out of the salon with my brand-new beautiful wig. Not a bad look—*If I do say so myself!* I thought Italy was a prime place to start wearing my wig, so I could get used to it and limit any novice wardrobe malfunctions.

The flight to Milan was a breeze. We were in business class, which provided a lot more room. I didn't sleep much. In between movies, I got up, stretched, and walked around a lot. I also massaged my legs under the compression stockings, in an effort to improve circulation in my legs. By the end of the flight, I saw three movies: *Miss Congeniality*, *Charlie's Angels*, and *Castaway*. I was feeling pretty good for only having an hour of sleep.

In Milan, we rented a car and drove to Lake Como. Or rather, my mom rented a car and she drove to Lake Como. I am not sure what kind of car it was, but it didn't fit much more than a suitcase in the trunk or in the small backseat. Luckily, Mom and I were small people; otherwise, we wouldn't have fit in it. The car didn't look particularly safe either. My petite Chrysler Sebring convertible could crush the tin can. The little car was a red piece of metal crap that I fondly called the Red Devil.

I didn't think about it until we were actually in the little car, but we were setting the stage for something mighty awful by having Mom drive and me navigate through the tiny towns of Italy in the Red Devil. Maybe I should have thought this part of the journey through a little more. This feeling increased dramatically after Mom started driving. I thought she was going to kill the engine by revving it so much. I don't know if there is such a thing, but it seemed like the Red Devil had a two-cylinder engine. I really should have considered the Red Devil in our planning.

We managed to make it to Lake Como without a blow-up. *Huge for us, considering the Red Devil, strange roads, strange signs, different language, jet lag, and short tempers.* We arrived at the exquisite entrance to the Villa D'este estate in awe of the amazing beauty of the resort grounds. As the Red Devil pulled up to the entrance, I noticed we weren't alone. The Red Devil pulled up next to Lamborghinis, Ferraris, and Rolls-Royces. While I was embarrassed about our new friend, the Red Devil, my mom was horrified. "Oh my God!" she screeched. "I am so humiliated! I can't believe we are at one of the nicest hotels in this Red Devil piece of shit!"

To the valet, "Please, take this car away and hide it. I think it is supposed to be eco-friendly or something." I don't think the valet cared.

Luckily, our room was ready *and* we received an upgrade! Our suite had a gorgeous view of Lake Como. We quickly checked out the room(s) and unpacked a little before heading out for lunch.

The adorable town of Cernobbio was a short walk from the hotel. We went to a quaint cafe that the concierge had recommended for nourishment. Both being exhausted, we went back to the hotel for a well-needed four hour nap.

When Mom woke me up, I had no idea where I was, what I was doing there, or what day it was. I was in such a deep sleep. I looked up at the gorgeous fourteen-foot ceiling and around the room. Wearing a white-and-gold luxurious robe, Mom was sitting on the bed with me, handing me a glass of champagne. I took the glass from her. With a big grin on her face, she grabbed the other glass and toasted, "Here's to our great Italian adventure!" *Clink.*

"Thanks, Mom. I can't tell you how much this trip means to me. For a while, I forgot all about cancer. It is definitely NOT top of mind, and I have you to thank for making that happen," I said as I wiped a tear off of my cheek and held her hand. "Look at me getting all emotional." *We were having a special moment.*

"All right. Let's get ready for dinner." Our moment was over.

I put on a cute dress and pashmina and took out my wig for its maiden voyage. We decided to stay local for dinner and went to the hotel restaurant, Veranda. The magnificent room had a beautiful view of Lake Como. As the sun set over the lake, I felt like I was in heaven. *This is just what I needed.*

We stopped by the bar for a closer before ending our first day. The piano singer was a bonus. *What a nice ending to a nice day! Cancer? What cancer?*

September 3, 2000

I was sleeping peacefully until I was suddenly awakened by my mom.

"Get up, lazy bones. You are going to sleep the day away. We have lots to do. Let's go."

She was opening the blinds. "Wow! What a view to wake up to. I would be happy sitting here all day, watching the lake and the boats," I responded.

"Come on. You can do that later. We are going to have a fun day! It's after 9:00. We need to leave around 10:00 for our trip to Lake Orta."

"All right, all right. I'm getting up," I said as I grabbed my journal and medications. The morning process began.

At 10:00 a.m., we had the Red Devil brought up for our drive to Lake Orta. Mom was the driver and I was the navigator. Again, I didn't think this was the best scenario, but she was not about to let me drive. She was the little lady in charge. I had her maps and directions all organized in my lap and was ready to go.

Lake Orta was a little over an hour away. It was supposed to be the most beautiful lake in Italy and less crowded than Lake Como. We had to take the tollway to get there. I was counting out the change when we pulled up to the booth.

"Hurry, Vicki, hurry! Give me that change!" she yelled in a panic.

"I'm getting it. Just a second."

"Just forget about it! I will use a credit card!"

Then she put the credit card in the slot. "I can't figure out what to do. It's in Italian. HELP!" she exclaimed, pressing any button she could. I jumped out of the car to inspect the booth. By the time I got around the car, she was yanking on the card trying to get it out, breathing heavily.

Meanwhile, the cars behind us were getting upset, honking their horns, and yelling in Italian. I tried to help but couldn't figure out how to get the card out. I waved over to an attendant, who took her time coming over to help, probably because she didn't want to deal with a hysterical lady. She didn't speak very much English but pushed some buttons and the card popped out. I gave the attendant some cash, and she let us go.

By this time, Mom was hyperventilating, sweating, and shaking. I asked her to pull over.

"Are you okay, Mom? Breathe slowly," I said as I rubbed her back and gave her water. Her breathing slowed down a bit.

"I don't know what came over me. I thought I was going to die," she muttered, still shaking.

"You are all right. I think you were having a panic attack."

"I guess so," she replied glumly while I hugged her.

"I tell you what. Why don't you let me drive and you can be the co-pilot, okay?"

"No! I'm driving," she said stubbornly.

Every once in a while I had to put my foot down. "Mom, you just had a panic attack and are still shaking. You are not driving anywhere. Now get out of the Red Devil and give me the keys." *Amazing! She is actually doing what I said!*

It was time for lunch by the time we got to Lake Orta. We ate at an outdoor cafe near the water. It was such a beautiful sunny day in the 70s. Besides the panic attack, we were having a lovely day. After lunch, we took a walk and ferry over to San Giulio Island. The island was filled with picturesque medieval buildings from the fourth through sixth centuries. Very cool.

Mom actually let me drive back to the hotel after our outing. *Hooray!* Funny, I used the word "let." We showered up and went to the terrace to listen to a combo play before dinner. With the sunset over the lake, my mom merrily over her panic attack, the glamorous hotel, my chardonnay, and my new wig, I was feeling incredible.

After dinner, we went back to the bar. Another combo was playing and people were dancing. We sat at a small table by the bar. Mom announced to me, "I am going to have a White Russian."

"Whoa! What's in a White Russian?"

"Vodka, Kahlua, and cream."

"What's in a Black Russian?"

"Vodka and Kahlua."

And just when Mom was sharing cocktail recipes with me, she exclaimed, "Oh God. Robert Duvall just walked in. Look to your left." And there he was, straight from the *Godfather*, Robert Duvall walking up to the bar.

"You go meet him. Walk up to the bar and order our drinks," I ordered her, wondering if he was single.

"Don't be silly. You do it."

"Just do it, Mom. Get a White Russian and I'll have a chardonnay," I prodded her.

Mom got up and walked over to the bar. She feebly tried to squeeze between a few men. "Well, come on up here, little lady," Robert Duvall said as he guided Mom to the bar. It kind of sounded like John Wayne. I couldn't hear the rest, but Mom had the biggest grin on her face. I was so happy to see it! He seemed like a gentleman.

She walked back to our table with the two drinks with that grin on her face. "And I didn't even have to pay for them."

"Are you kidding me? Did Robert Duvall pay for our drinks?"

"No, but the guy next to him did!" she cheered.

What fun! She actually met Robert Duvall. Wouldn't it be nice if he asked her to dance. Or the other guy. But, no. They left.

As I went to sleep that night, I thought about how grateful I was to be in Italy. I was feeling tired, but even my limbs felt better. *Maybe my cancer is going away?*

September 4, 2000

I told Mom not to wake me up. I knew ahead of time that I was going to need sleep. I woke up naturally around ten in the morning. Mom left me a note to meet her at the pool, so I hung out in my fancy robe and started my process. For some reason, the process goes by faster when you have somewhere great to go.

I met Mom down at the floating pool. I had never seen a floating pool before. It was an actual pool and pool deck floating in Lake Como. We spent the day there sunbathing, having lunch, and kayaking. It was so cool. When you got hot you could jump in the pool or the lake.

I took a nap in the afternoon. Not only was I tired, but my nausea was kicking in, so I slept with the wastebasket next to me. When I woke up, I felt much better. We had our nightly pre- and post-cocktail at the hotel and ventured into the town for dinner. I found myself looking for Robert Duvall everywhere. I really wanted him to hook up with my mom. *Wouldn't that be fun!*

September 5, 2000

We needed to get up little earlier than usual due to a boat tour we took on Lake Como to Bellagio. I was dragging but made myself hang in there. It was, yet again, another perfect day in Italy.

The boat ride across Lake Como was exhilarating. Our driver pointed out famous mansions on the lake, such as Versace and Heinz. Bellagio was a picturesque town and interesting to walk around and shop. We had lunch and took the boat back to the Villa D'este for an afternoon spa day. No nap was required.

September 6, 2000

Mom and I had an amazing breakfast on the terrace. It was our only real breakfast at the Villa D'este. Surprisingly, I ran into a friend of mine from the corporation at breakfast. *What a small world.* He had heard about my cancer through the grapevine, so we talked about that and the changes at the corporation. It was fun catching up.

After breakfast, Mom and I took a walk through the gardens on the property, which was something we had been intending on doing since we got there. The gardens were gorgeous and pristine. I couldn't imagine how many people they had keeping the gardens so perfect. I never saw anyone taking care of the gardens the whole time we had been staying there. *Maybe little leprechauns come by at night to trim and water the bushes and flowers.*

We checked out and drove the Red Devil to the airport in Milan. It was time to say goodbye to the Red Devil and hello to a carless Positano. We took a flight from Milan to Naples and had Luigi drive us from to the San Pietro hotel in Positano. Thank God we didn't rent a car! The Red Devil would not have made it around the hairpin turns with either of us driving.

Luigi was awesome in a few respects. First of all, he was a great driver. Second, he helped relax my mom during the drive. Mom had another panic attack in the airport. She was extra nervous about finding our luggage, finding Luigi, and driving to the hotel. I found this unusual, because I had never seen her so insecure. She was always on top of things and self-assured. The only other time I had seen her so insecure was when my dad was dying. I found myself jumping in and taking control in these situations.

Coming from one amazing hotel and going to another, we were living the high-life. Mom was really treating me to a special trip. While the Villa D'este had its own beauty on Lake Como, the San Pietro had a different kind of beauty to it. The hotel was built in a cliff overlooking the magnificent Mediterranean. There were gorgeous paths along the flowery cliff leading to the rooms with incredible views. It didn't seem like there were that many rooms in the hotel. The restaurant was on top of the cliff, and the beach was accessible by an elevator inside the cliff that took you down to the sea.

On the first night, we had dinner outside on top of the cliff with the best view of the hotel. There was a piano singer that we listened to during dinner. Since the hotel was exclusive and quaint, we got to know the other visitors from around the world as well as the staff. There were three Luigis and a Casanova. It was pretty easy to distinguish them. When in doubt, it's Luigi. We crashed early due to an exhausting day.

September 7, 2000

I continued wearing a baseball cap during the day and my wig at night. My head got to breathe while we were in the hotel room. We ordered room service for breakfast on our terrace, so I put my cap on. While we ate on our terrace, we watched the sea and the yachts. There was one huge yacht, in particular, that we watched while it was parking in front of our hotel. It was fascinating.

After breakfast, we went down to the beach for a swim. The Mediterranean was therapeutic. Just floating in the water, I felt like my cancer was exiting my body. I decided to believe that the sea was making me better, whether it was or it wasn't.

The hotel used the elevator as a service elevator to bring whatever we needed to the lounge chairs. Casanova brought us lunch and started flirting with me, which was flattering. Casanova was a casanova—very fitting. He called me Victoria (Beektoria). The service was phenomenal. *I could live here forever!*

The hotel arranged a private boat for us and another couple to take a tour of the Amalfi Coast. We saw Sophia Loren's house and stopped at a beach for a swim. We had dinner back at the hotel. Mom wanted to see the piano player again. So, we did.

"I love the way the pianist tinkles the keys," Mom told me.

"What?" I asked with a smirk.

"I love the way the pianist tinkles the keys," she repeated more loudly, so the room could hear. Mom speaks loudly as it is, and when she repeats herself, watch out!

I couldn't contain myself any longer. I leaned over and let her know, "Mom, a pianist tickles the keys. He does not pee on them." We both laughed, and even got a few chuckles out of one of the Luigis.

September 8, 2000

Our only day of rain occurred on the day we had a tour of Pompeii. It was kind of a bummer, but we made the best of it. A couple from Louisville joined us for the day. We were making friends left and right at the hotel.

Pompeii in the rain was still really cool. You walk through this ancient city that was destroyed by twenty feet of volcanic ash in AD 79. The ash preserved the city, and we were able to see what life was like almost two thousand years ago. The whorehouse was actually the highlight of the tour.

The history lesson is over.

Mom and I went back to the hotel and took a nap while it rained. Once again, we had dinner at the hotel with our new friends, Casanova, the three Luigis, and the pianist. We didn't all actually eat together. Mom and I ate together but chatted up our new peeps.

September 9, 2000

I could get used to the breakfast room service and view off of our terrace. Each morning Casanova or one of the Luigis would bring it to us. Of course, we were living the leisure life of having breakfast in our robes and me in my cap.

We went to the beach in the morning and to the town of Positano in the afternoon. The town was adorable. We shopped and had dinner on a rooftop overlooking the Mediterranean. Instead of hanging out in town, we went back to our hotel bar to our new friends and pianist. It was our last night, and we needed a proper send-off.

September 10, 2000

Our last morning at the San Pietro included having our final breakfast on our terrace. We were packing when Casanova came to the door with our breakfast. I went to open the door wigless and capless.

"Buongiorno, Casanova!" I greeted him with a smile. He froze. Casanova's jaw dropped as he looked at me as though I had three heads. I had no idea I was wigless and capless and couldn't figure out what was wrong with him. The suave Casanova was speechless. He had been flirting with me for three days and had no idea I was bald!

"Ah, Buongiorno, Victoria." He swiftly put the tray on the table and left the room. Mom and I looked at each other and cracked up.

Mom and I took a cab to Sorrento and spent two nights in an old monastery before going home. It was interesting staying in a monastery—quite different from San Pietro for sure. We spent the day at Capri and then flew home. What an incredible trip we had. It was just what the doctor ordered!

September 14, 2000

My cousin Jamie was in town on business from Tucson and stayed with us for a few days. She was such a sweetheart. She took me to my eighth chemo, which was either halfway finished or, preferably, two-thirds of the way done. My WBC was a low 900, so the doctor ordered Neupogen shots for me to take before the next chemo. I thought they told me I couldn't have chemo if my WBC was below 1500, but we continued with the chemo process anyway.

Italy was such a nice distraction for me. Now I was back in the world of blood tests, IV drips, shots, CT scans, etc. It was kind of depressing, but I had Jamie to keep me company for the day, which was an enjoyable distraction.

I set the chemo process expectations with Jamie and the process began. Jamie seemed nervous about the process, but she wanted to be there for me. About an hour into the process, I began to taste the chemo. Yuck. The metallic taste made me sick. I felt like I was swimming in a pool of poison and couldn't get out. Goodbye Italy. Hello reality.

September 16, 2000

Jamie was very happy to be a part of "Team Vicki." She had been supportive from afar sending flowers and cards and an occasional phone call, which was really appreciated. Being there in person helped even more. She even stayed and went to "Light the Night" with "Team Vicki."

I slept in and rested in preparation for Light the Night. Julie signed us up as "Team Vicki." Light the Night was a fundraiser for the Leukemia and Lymphoma Society downtown in Grant Park from 5:00 p.m. to 8:00 p.m. My team consisted of Julie, Jamie, Sharon, Heather, Heather Mac, Cate, Sue, Robin, Karen, Colleen, and me. Julie reserved a wheelchair for me, so we did the mile walk together, as a team, marching Vicki along Lake Michigan with balloons flying everywhere. There were also luminaries lit up all along the lake. It was actually a really fun time with some of my closest friends, even if I was feeling tired and queasy. "Team Vicki" raised $10,600 for the Leukemia and Lymphoma Society. I had an unforgettable time with supportive friends, and raised money for the cause. Win/win!

September 27, 2000

I hung out in bed for a while thinking about stuff after I woke up. Stuff consisted of my illness, my friends, my family, my job, and my millennium. It had been a month or so since I took my leave of absence. I was so lucky I was able to stop working, because I couldn't imagine working the way I was feeling queasy and tired all of the time. Not to mention, chemo brain. I wasn't myself anymore. I could still turn on the charm and smile, but underneath I was a body full of poison ready to explode. I considered the fact that I could be flammable. I should ask the doctor about that one.

I had no idea if I was going back to the start-up or somewhere else altogether. Frankly, I didn't care. I just wanted to get rid of the cancer and feel better. My friends and family had been very supportive, and I was extra grateful for them. I thought about my goals for the year and how I had failed miserably at my millennium goals (health, men, career). I had even gained back the weight I had lost. I couldn't understand how I had gained the weight back, because I was sick as a dog and not eating much.

I thought about how I looked different when I looked in the mirror. Obviously, my hair looked different, but my skin color was different (purplish), my face was swollen, my neck was swollen, and my stomach was swollen. Apparently, the swelling was Cushing's syndrome caused by steroids.

I decided to focus on the positive and write down all of the things that I was grateful for in my journal. I wrote and wrote and wrote. Then I wrote down all of the things that make Vicki happy. I wrote and wrote and wrote. After I finished this kumbaya moment with myself, I was ready to start my day and my process. I was quite satisfied with this moment and decided to have these moments more often. Wash out the negative thoughts and be grateful.

I went downstairs for my Raisin Bran and greeted Mom with an extra spring in my step.

"What's up with you?" she said, noticing my extra spring.

"Now is that any way to greet your darling daughter in the morning? Good morning, mother dear!"

"Good morning, Vicki. You seem like you are in a good mood. Are you feeling better?"

"I guess I am. I gave myself an attitude adjustment this morning."

"Well, whatever you did, I want some of it!"

I went upstairs and called Kristen. She had called me a few times, and I needed to get back with her. "Hey, Kris. Sorry it has taken me a while to get back to you."

"No problem. I just wanted to catch up with you. How are you feeling?"

"I'm okay. I am having a CT scan today. I can't wait to see what's going on with these tumors. Hey, you never told me about your raft trip."

"Good luck with the scan. Please let me know when you know the results. I'm assuming Mom told you about the trip?"

"Well, yeah, but I want to hear your version."

"Ah, yes. Well, she did pretty well with the cousins. She kept up pretty well. She even went kayaking a few times. Did she tell you she almost died?"

"Why, yes, she did. It sounded terrible."

"She probably totally exaggerated. It was a class-one rapid, and even Kirby was kayaking down it. It was about one and a half feet deep. She fell out and was completely hysterical. All she had to do was stand up and she would have been fine. She just kept yelling that she was dying. I kind of felt sorry for her. The cousins were all howling, and the guides were rushing over to help her."

"Ah...she *did* exaggerate. Maybe the trip was too much for her."

"She was fine. She should have stayed on Cleopatra's Barge."

And from then on, Mom has shared the story of how she almost died with anyone who would listen. I listened patiently, knowing the truth. My cousins always cracked up when she talked about it.

After breakfast and my conversation with Kristen, I went to the hospital for a CT scan and Neupogen shot. I was looking forward to both. I wanted to see if my tumors had shrunk, and the Neupogen shot was going to give me more white blood cells to fight infection. Both were easy peasy. I felt like I had had a million CT scans, like I could do them in my sleep. The Neupogen shot was no biggie also. Those were my duties of the day until dinner club.

I came home and took a nap. I wanted to be at my best for dinner club. Most of the girls had not seen my wig yet, and I wanted to look my best, even if I had a fat face. Sue picked me up and we went to Highwood for dinner. Ten of us were there that night. It was usually between six and eleven people at dinner club, so it was a pretty good showing.

Everyone liked my wig. Some liked it better than my own hair. Well, they didn't actually say that, but the way they went on about my wig, I assumed they liked it better than my real hair.

We were having a wonderful time talking, when someone noticed Michael Jordan sitting at the bar. I knew he didn't live far from there but was surprised to see him in public. By this time, I had had a few glasses of wine and was feeling somewhat assertive.

I got up from the table, marched right over to Michael, and stuck out my hand. "Hi, Michael! I'm Vicki."

Michael smiled his Michael smile, which is priceless. He shook my hand and introduced me to his friend. Wow! His hand was huge! I expected it to be big, but it was *really* big. He was friendly and inquired about our group. I explained our dinner club.

I couldn't help myself. "You know, Michael, my friend Heather over there played golf with you at Skokie about eight years ago, and you guys got rained out. She was beating you at the time. I think you guys should have a rematch."

Michael grinned. "Hmmm. I don't remember."

His buddy chimed in. "You do know you are talking to the most competitive person in the world."

"Of course I know that! I also think he doesn't want to back down from a challenge. My friend Heather is very competitive too." I motioned toward Heather. "Heather, come over here!"

Heather was hesitant to move. Michael motioned. "Come on over, Heather!" Just then, I actually thought I had a shot at getting a match put together. Begrudgingly, Heather came over.

Michael stuck out his hand, "Nice to meet you, Heather."

"Hi, Michael."

"You know you two already met," I clarified. And, of course, I had to brag, "Heather won State in golf and played at ASU."

"Come on, Vicki," Heather tried to make me stop, but there wasn't any stopping me, once I got started.

"Well, congratulations. You must be great at golf."

"Thank you." She was really embarrassed.

I kept pushing, "Heather, I was reminding Michael about when you played golf together. I think you guys should have a rematch. My money's on you."

"Oh, Vicki, don't be silly. Don't bother him with that," she responded.

I think Michael's friend was getting annoyed with the conversation. "Sorry, ladies. It was nice to meet you, but Michael doesn't have time for this."

"Let's leave it between Michael and Heather." I thought maybe that was the best way to leave it. Peace out. I walked away thinking that Michael couldn't resist a challenge from cute blonde Heather. I went back to our group and filled them in on our conversation.

Heather talked with Michael and his friend for a few minutes and returned to our table. My inquiring mind wanted to know, "Well, tell us! What happened?"

"Nothing. We just talked about golf," she said.

"Are you going to have a rematch?" I wanted to know.

"No. We didn't even talk about it."

I was so bummed. I teed it up and everything. Oh well…

The action was over, and so was dinner club. Sue drove me home to Mom's.

September 28, 2000

Chemo Day! Colleen picked me up for chemo. She was also one of my high school friends. I was excited and nervous to know what my CT scan revealed. This put me in a quiet mood.

My blood count was borderline, so we went ahead with the chemo process. I gave Colleen my usual warning, which she already knew by chatting with the other girls. I was getting anxious about my CT scan results. "Daniela, are my CT scan results back?" I asked as she was plugging the IV into my port like it was an outlet.

"Yes. They are back. Dr. Kim will come see you, when she has time."

"Okay. Tell her I am anxious to get them back."

"Oh, she knows."

I think Dr. Kim likes me as much as I like her. It was a bit confusing to me why someone like her would go into oncology if she had no compassion for her patients. I could tell she thought I was a complainer and a wimp. She gave me these looks like, "What do you have to complain about? Other patients are a lot worse off." She also seemed annoyed about my extremity issues. It was like she thought they were not her problem and outside her purview. Maybe if she had gone through something similar, she would have more compassion. I started to complain to Colleen about her and then caught myself.

"Sorry, Colleen. Maybe I *am* a complainer. I just wish that she pretended to care."

"It seems to me that you probably have a right to complain."

"Well, she is supposed to be a very good doctor, so I will deal with it."

We watched TV, and I fell asleep to be awakened by my favorite person. "Good morning, Vicki." Dr. Kim was in the house. I tried to clear my head and get out my list of questions from my journal.

"Hi, Dr. Kim. How are you?"

"Fine, thanks. How are you feeling?"

"Groggy and nauseous. This is my friend, Colleen."

"Hi, Colleen. I hope you don't mind leaving the room while I examine Vicki."

"No problem. I will go to the cafeteria. I'll get you a Diet Coke, Vicki," Colleen replied as she left the room.

Dr. Kim examined me while I became more and more nervous about the news.

"Do you have my CT scan results?" I asked.

"Why yes, I do. Your thoracic tumor is now scar tissue, and the tumor by your heart is now 2 x 4 cm," she said with a smile.

I smiled. "That's good news, right?"

"Well, yes. It is, but not good enough yet."

"What does that mean?"

"We will check it again in two months. If it is not gone, we will continue with the chemo for another two months and maybe follow it up with radiation. Also, you need to continue with the Neupogen shots to keep up your WBC."

Okay. I guess that is good news. It isn't bad news. As long as we are going in the right direction, that is good news. Yes. This is good news. I have decided.

Colleen came back. I gave her the good news. "My tumors have shrunk! One is gone and the other is a lot smaller!"

Colleen beamed. "That's great news, Vicki! I am so happy for you!"

We finished up the chemo, and Colleen took me home. When we pulled up to Mom's house, I got a surge of emotion and hugged Colleen. "Thank you so much for taking me to chemo. I really appreciate it." And I started sobbing in her arms.

Mystified in my sudden mood change, Colleen hugged me back, "It's my pleasure, Vicki. I am happy to help. Please let me know whatever you need. I want to help you."

"Just being here, you are." And I got out of the car, gathered myself together, and went into Mom's house.

I told Mom the news. She had a similar reaction as I did. "It's definitely an improvement," she said as we discussed it. I went and took a nap before dinner.

Chapter Ten

October 2000: My Wake and Bake

> "Hard things will happen to us. We will recover. We will learn from it. We will grow more resilient because of it."
>
> — Taylor Swift

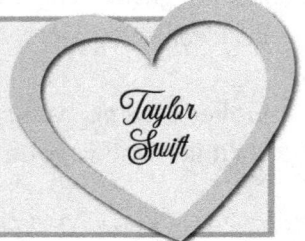

October 1, 2000

Mom continued her dedication toward keeping Vicki entertained by taking me to my aunt's cottage to hang out and see the fall colors, just the two of us. My mom's sister, Aunt Nancy, had a winterized cottage on Long Lake in Phelps, Wisconsin. We had visited there every summer growing up and a few winters too. Mom drove the six hours to get there, while I slept most of the way. Every once in a while she would wake me up and tell me to look at the beautiful leaves on the trees. The trees became more and more dense as we drove north. There were also more and more pine trees. I always knew when we were getting close to the cottage when we drove through Eagle River, the metropolis, tourist trap, and snowmobile capital of the world.

The cottage was in the middle of a really long lake, hence the name. There were only a few cottages on the lake, so it felt like your very own personal lake. As we drove down the long, winding, rock driveway, I thought about all of the happy memories I have had at Aunt Nancy's cottage water skiing, boating, and playing in the woods. Those were the days!

The weather was typical, a high of seventy degrees. It was sunny and beautiful as we looked out at the bright reflection of the leaves on the calm lake. The cottage sat on a hill, so it was a tough walk down to the dock and back, especially in the condition I was in. That was the first thing I did. Mom warned me, "What goes down, must come up! I hope you can make it! I can't carry you back up!"

Of course, super-Vicki responded, "Don't worry about me!" I sat on the dock for about a half an hour and started the trek back up to the cottage. Okay, so Mom was right. I huffed and puffed and took about five breaks on the way up. *I hate it when Mom's right.*

We made a fire in the huge stone fireplace and got cozy. At Aunt Nancy's cottage, we did not watch TV. We read books, listened to music, and played games.

I took out my Harry Potter book, put on Simon and Garfunkel, and read my book in front of the fire with a glass of wine. I was in heaven, right along with Mom. This was right up her alley. We made chicken and broccoli for dinner. That was right up my alley.

October 2, 2000

I woke up to a fresh chill in the air due to my window being cracked open. At first, I had no idea where I was. Then it set in. I went back to sleep with a smile on my face.

Mom woke me up around ten in the morning. "Get up, lazy bones!" *I think I am allowed to be lazy bones.* I didn't move. She came into the room. "Are you going to sleep all day?"

"Okay, I am getting up!" The process started, and I headed into the kitchen for my Raisin Bran.

After we ate, we went on a walk. It was a beautiful fall day with the leaves at their prime. I kept noticing how fresh the air was. On a day-to-day basis, I never noticed that the air was polluted in Chicago. You really notice it when you go to a clean environment. You also really notice the bright stars. Life was different in the north woods.

After our walk, we hung out, made lunch, and read some more. Life was simple in the north woods. I took a nap and got ready for our big night out at the supper club, the Tijuana. *Who knew that the best ribs in the United States, and maybe the world, are in a small supper club in the north woods?*

The Tijuana was similar to a lot of the supper clubs in the area. It was an old log cabin with several rooms decorated with stuffed animals, fish, and birds: a bear, an owl, a few deer, a fox, walleye, bass, etc. I am not sure how long it had been there, but I had been going there my whole life. The difference between the Tijuana and other supper clubs was the ribs. I had never gotten anything there but ribs. Even in my sick condition and lack of appetite, I ate the ribs. And the best part was taking some home for leftovers. Yum.

We went home and crashed. It was 8:00 p.m. Actually, Mom probably stayed up to read for a few hours.

October 3, 2000

Today was our big day out. We went to the Indian reservation about a half an hour away by Watersmeet, Michigan. Lac Vieux Desert had both a casino and a golf course. Mom and I brought our golf clubs with us and played. Well, she played, and I cheered her on. The golf course was in unusually great shape. Mom and I assumed it was because the proceeds from the casino went into the golf course, making it so incredible to play.

I spent most of my time in the golf cart, getting out to chip and putt here and there. We made it fun by betting on the closest to the pin on chips and putts.

After golf, we made our way to the casino. It looked like a big warehouse on the outside. It smelled like an ashtray on the inside. I think we were there during the off-season, because there were only a few of us in the whole place. There was no way the casino could support the golf course with this puny crowd. It had a bar, a restaurant, and a large number of the typical games. Neither of us being big betters, we found a novice blackjack table and lost some money. Then, we went to the slots and lost some money. Finally, we went to the roulette table and lost some money. After that, we called it a day.

On the way back to the cottage we went to another supper club. This time it was filled with mounted championship walleye and bass. I bet taxidermy was one of the biggest professions in the area. Seeing all of the stuffed fish, both Mom and I were convinced we had to order fish. We sat down, and the server gave us each a scoop of ice cream. We thought that was kind of strange. "Why are you giving us ice cream?" Mom just had to know.

"That's not ice cream, that's cheese," the server informed us. Mom and I looked at each other and burst out laughing. Yes, we were indeed in cheeseland.

I intended on ordering fish, but once I got the menu, I couldn't help ordering the prime rib for $12. I couldn't believe it was only $12. *Who has a $12 prime rib and actually makes money on it?* It had to be horrible.

The prime rib was delivered to our table, and it was the best prime rib I had ever had. And I wasn't even hungry. *You gotta love supper clubs!*

Mom and I drove by a herd of deer on the way home. *I love Wisconsin!*

October 4-5, 2000

Mom and I had a lazy last day, reading in the cottage, going on a walk, and playing games.

Mom drove home while I slept again. Oh, and I puked. Luckily, she pulled over in the nick of time. I apologized for being such a lousy driving partner.

October 12, 2000

I used to look forward to Chemo Day, because it was one step closer to being in remission. I no longer felt that way. It was becoming harder and harder to keep my chin up. Karen took me to chemo again. I didn't have to give my spiel this time. When she came and picked me up, she was so full of energy, it both energized me and made me sick at the same time.

It was only Karen's second time taking me, but she acted like a regular. "Hi, Daniela, how are you?"

"Good. Nice to see you again," Daniela replied, wondering who the heck Karen was.

"You remember Karen? Don't you?" I chimed in.

"Of course!"

No she didn't.

I guess the Neupogen shots had been working, because my blood counts were okay. Daniela plugged me in, and away we went. Karen brought a book this time, and I slept. The TV didn't even come on. They woke me up for my meeting with Dr. Kim, who informed me that she didn't think I had a paraneoplastic syndrome and that it was the chemo making me aching, throbbing, weak, and numb. I was in no mood to argue.

I was sick as a dog on the way home, taking a barf bag with me. I was thinking that maybe I shouldn't have friends take me to chemo anymore. I didn't like them seeing me like that. Hopefully, I had only a few more chemos. *If I am getting better, why am I feeling worse?* I understood it, I thought, but it still didn't make sense.

October 14, 2000

I developed a new habit! I started taking baths with *Harry Potter*! *Harry Potter* was all the rage, and I joined in on it. It was a very large book but was easy to read in Mom's very large tub. It was also an easy read for my chemo brain.

In the past, I had always liked taking relaxing baths every now and then. This fall, they became an important part of my healing journey. Taking baths especially helped my throbbing limbs. No one told me to do it, I just started doing it. I usually stayed in the tub for an hour, but sometimes I would get wrapped up in my book, and time would get away from me. Every once in a while Mom would yell, "Get out of the tub, Vicki! You will be a wrinkly mess!" I thought, *I was a wrinkly mess a half an hour ago.*

Anyway, I took my daily bath and put on my sweats. Mom was getting ready to go out to dinner with some friends at the club. I hung out in her bedroom chatting with her. Suddenly, my nausea followed through, true to its form, and I puked in her wastebasket. She came out of her bathroom and saw me hugging her wastebasket on the floor.

"Oh, Vicki. I am so sorry. What can I do for you?" She seemed very worried.

"I don't think there is anything you can do. I took my anti-nausea medication. I don't know what else we can do." None of the nausea medication worked. I had tried them all. I was so weak, gripping the wastebasket. It was my life raft. The room was spinning. I tried to focus but couldn't.

"I can't leave you like this."

"There isn't anything you can do."

"Well, let me get you to bed."

"I like it on the floor," I said in my misery. I didn't want to move. I didn't think I could get up. *Maybe I can sleep here?*

She finished getting ready and insisted, "Okay, time to get up." She helped me into my bedroom with me gripping the wastebasket. She was so small, she could hardly handle my weight leaning on her. She put the phone next to me. "Now, do not hesitate to call the club if you get any worse or need anything."

For some reason, I remember this bout of nausea in particular, because I actually did puke and was extra miserable from my head to my toes. The chemo poison really was poisoning me. I no longer had blood in my veins. Just poison. I was no longer Vicki. I was another person who I didn't know and didn't like. I wanted the old Vicki back. I wasn't sure whether she would ever come back or what she would be like, if she did come back.

October 15, 2000

I actually felt better in the morning. I am not sure why. I started my process and went down to breakfast. Mom was there, reading her paper.

"Good morning! How are you feeling?"

"Better. I think I can eat my Raisin Bran."

"Good. Last night, Sandi told me that you should probably smoke marijuana. Maybe it will help the pain and nausea?" This came out of left field. I was not expecting my mom to encourage me to smoke pot.

"Really? I guess it couldn't hurt." Actually, it was a great idea!

"I want you to call Hugh and get some marijuana."

"I'll figure out where to get it. Don't worry about it."

"No. I want you to call Hugh right now," she ordered me. Then, we argued about it for the next ten minutes, and I called Hugh. She always won. I don't even know why I tried.

I was really annoyed. Mom was sitting right next to me as I dialed. I was hoping he didn't answer, but he did. I felt like a child. *My mommy told me I have to call you.*

"Hi, Hugh. It's Vicki."

"Hey, Vicki, how are you doing?"

"Okay. I am pretty nauseous, and I was wondering if you knew where I could get some pot. I thought it might help me." Mom was trying to listen in, and I had to get up and leave the room.

"Oh, geez Vicki. I have no idea where to get it. I can check around for you, but I can't promise you anything."

Then, from the peanut gallery in the other room, my mom called out, "Ask him if his brother can get it!"

"No. My brother can't get it either. You know he hasn't smoked in years," Hugh responded. "I'll let you know if I can find some."

Well, that was embarrassing. I reassured Mom that I could find some and left it at that.

October 25, 2000

We had dinner club in Glenview, which was easier for the suburbanites, including me now. Sue picked me up. As I got in the car, she gave me a Christmas cookie tin. As I accepted the cookies, I thanked her. "Thanks, Sue! That was nice of you."

"Ah, Vicki. Those aren't cookies."

I opened the tin and was pleasantly surprised when I saw a bag of pot, a one-hitter and a pipe. Christmas came early!

"Ah-ha! It was very nice of you!"

"I was told that stuff was really strong, so watch out!"

Whether I liked it or not, I was about to become a pot smoker.

October 26, 2000

Heather picked me up for chemo. We hadn't had a chance to catch up in a while. We were about to spend most of the day together.

"So, Hugh told me you asked him to get you some pot," she blurted out.

"Oh my gosh. Hysterical. My mom made me call him, because she thought he could find it. I still have to apologize to him."

"Don't worry about it. Did you find some?"

"Actually, Sue gave me some last night. I haven't had any yet. I am hoping it helps my nausea, because it is really bad now. Maybe I will try it tonight. Oh, and sorry about the Michael Jordan thing, again. I know I embarrassed you, but I couldn't help it."

"No problem. It was fun talking to him, again. I am sure he remembered me."

Chemo went by, as usual, except this time I had a puke bag next to me ready to go. I scheduled my next CT scan and Neupogen shots. *God, I hope I am done soon!*

Heather drove me home, and I took a nap before dinner. Mom woke me up. "It is time to wake and bake! Vicki, you need to get up and smoke your pot before dinner!" she yelled up the stairs. Half asleep, I giggled. *I can't believe my mom is ordering me to smoke pot.*

"Okay. Where do you want me to smoke it?" I asked.

"Why don't you go down to the laundry room and smoke it. Dinner is in a half an hour."

I got up and took my cookie tin to the laundry room in the basement, thinking it was a strange place to do it, but whatever. I wasn't sure what I was doing. I took the one-hitter and shoved some flakes in it. The stuff smelled like a skunk. It reeked. I was scared I was going to puke as I inhaled, so I did it over the sink. I took one drag and started coughing profusely. Okay, maybe I took too much. I took another drag and still coughed. It was going to take me a while to become a real pot smoker.

I left the pot in the laundry room, which now smelled like a skunk. I went upstairs to the kitchen where Mom was cooking dinner. Suddenly, I was hungry! I couldn't remember the last time I was actually hungry. Wow! I was a new woman!

"Mom, I'm hungry!" I announced with delight.

"That's wonderful, Vicki!"

I loved my dinner. This was magical. *Why did it take me so long to figure this out?*

"Great dinner, Mom!"

"Go smoke some more, when you are done." And I went back downstairs to continue my life-changing new habit.

Chapter Eleven
November 2000: My Barbados

> "Optimism is a happiness magnet. If you stay positive, good things and good people will be drawn to you."
>
> — Mary Lou Retton

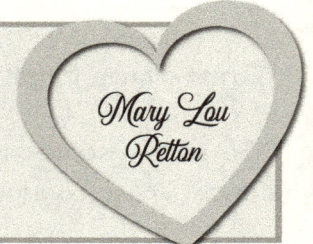

November 6, 2000

I thought maybe I would go downtown to make sure my house was still standing. I had to be there on the 7th to vote, anyway.

Yes, my house was still standing. I collected the mail, which had dispersed all over the floor and blocked my entrance. I missed my place, but it felt very cold and lonely. I was lucky to have Mom's to stay at in my time of need. She would probably need me someday too. What comes around, goes around...

November 7, 2000

Election Day! I wanted to make sure I voted, because it is important to vote, but it is tough in the state of Illinois, if you are Republican. Illinois is pretty much a Democratic state. There are a number of ways my vote did count, even if my vote for Bush didn't matter. I went to the school down the street to vote after I was finished with my process. I was one of the only people voting. I guess I hit a good time?

The rest of the day I napped, cleaned, washed my clothes, and re-packed for going back to Mom's. I kept tabs on the election results as I was doing my chores. Day became night, and the election was extremely close. I watched the TV from my bed and was in and out of sleep. I was dazed and confused. They called the election for Al Gore at one point. Shit! Then they called the election for George Bush. Yes! Then it went to a recall due to Florida being won by Bush by a fraction of a percentage. I was so confused. Little did I know that it would end up in the Supreme Court and have a "hanging chad" controversy. I will always remember that night, floating in and out of sleep, wondering who would be the next president.

November 9, 2000

Sue picked me up for chemo. Luckily, I got to go to chemo a little later because I couldn't see Dr. Kim until 4:00 p.m. I didn't like going first thing in the morning. It rushed my morning process, which had a few more steps now due to my becoming a pothead. Wake and bake was the new step that I added to the beginning of the process, which allowed me to get through the process with ease. I thought about telling Dr. Kim I was a pothead and decided not to.

I didn't want her to cramp my style. I had finally found something that helped my nausea, no thanks to her.

"Hey Sue! I have to tell you how amazing you are!" I greeted Sue.

"Well, thanks, Vick. You finally noticed?"

"The pot you got me is helping my quality of life so much! I can't thank you enough!"

"It's supposed to be good stuff."

"Well, I wouldn't know, but it *is* working."

"That's what I am here for. I am your dealer now."

I hit the trifecta during my chemo drip—sleep, cry, puke. So fun!

After I finished puking, Dr. Kim came in, I grabbed my journal, and Sue went to the cafeteria. We discussed my upcoming Barbados trip and the all-important CT scan that I needed to take to determine whether I was done with chemo or not. She didn't seem to understand how important it was for me to get out of town again.

"You are throwing off the chemo schedule by a week," she informed me.

"If I am supposed to be finished with chemo, one week shouldn't matter," I pleaded.

"I guess we can do it. Why don't you have the CT scan right before you leave for Barbados, and then we can meet right after you get home."

"So I will be wondering the whole time if I am done or not?"

"Why don't you think positively and assume you are finished? It can be a celebration trip."

"Good idea. I will do that."

Besides Barbados, we discussed my nausea, without discussing my pothead status. I informed her that I was having problems breathing. She listened to my lungs and scheduled a pulmonary function test. I gave up on discussing my aching limbs, because she viewed that as complaining about something that she was not responsible for. We called it a day.

November 17, 2000

I had my all-important scan today. As I was being scanned, I wished my cancer away. I hoped that the radiation I received during the scan finalized the destruction of the tumors.

November 18, 2000

I tried to get a good night's sleep, but I was too excited for the trip. I was worried about my alarm going off at 4:30 a.m. I didn't want to be late and get the wrath of Barbara. That would be a bad way to start the trip. I would rather start the trip tired than get the wrath of Barbara.

I had to leave my one-hitter at home along with my bag of pot. I didn't want to get caught with it going through customs. I was going to miss my magic wand and potion. Hopefully, the sea, sand, and sun would compensate for the missing one hitter.

We had to fly through Miami to get to Barbados. The trip took about nine hours to get there, but it was worth it. We arrived at the Colony Club in the afternoon, made a pit stop to check out the room, and went directly to the swim-up bar for our welcome drink. We were greeted by Laverne and Shirfeelia, bartenders extraordinaire.

"Barbara, Vicki! Welcome back!" said Shirfeelia with a smile and a wave.

"We missed you two," added Laverne.

"Hi, Shirfeelia! Hi, Laverne! It is so good to be back!" Mom said.

"Hello, ladies," I said.

We ordered two Barbados punches, and Mom got right down to business. "Ladies, unfortunately I have bad news to share. Vicki has cancer, is taking chemo, and is not feeling well." *Way to go, Mom. How embarrassing.*

"Oh Vicki, I am sorry you are sick. We will make you feel much better," Shirfeelia responded sympathetically.

Laverne added, "You poor thing! Let us know what we can do for you. But you look good."

"Thanks. Don't worry about me. I am just happy to be here with you, in this beautiful weather. I'm okay, but I won't be water skiing."

Shirfeelia shared sincerely, "You can always water ski when you are better. For now, relax and have a wonderful trip."

And that is what we did.

November 19, 2000

We slept until the sun leaked into our room and the waterfall outside our room turned on. It was 8:00 a.m. and time to start our day. Mom went to go save our chairs, while I completed my process. It was a gorgeous day, and I couldn't wait to take advantage of it.

Sometimes we sat on the beach, and sometimes we sat by the pool. This morning was a beach morning. The sand was a pristine white sand leading into an alluring blue sea. The large swimming area was roped off, and a raft floated a few lengths out for swimmers to enjoy. A watersports hut was at one end providing everything from snorkel equipment to sailboats. Typically, I was the first and last one to water ski each day. I would miss that this year. Instead, I swam out to the raft to enjoy the sun on the raft. I was covered with sunscreen from head to toe and wearing one of my sun-drenched baseball caps.

Mom picked out two great lounge chairs positioned perfectly for the Caribbean Sea view, sun, and cabana boy. Well, Andrew wasn't exactly a boy. I would have put him around fifty. Andrew was our man. Andrew was our man of many words.

"Good morning, Andrew!" I greeted him. I think he mumbled "good morning" back.

"Mom and I are back in town for the week," I told him. He smiled.

"It's nice to see you," I added. He nodded and smiled.

"Can you save these chairs for us every morning?" I asked him.

"Sure." He nodded and smiled.

And we were in business. We tipped Andrew pretty well. He seemed happy with it. It was hard to tell.

We had lunch by the grotto pool near the swim-up bar. It was a beautiful pool winding back by all of the rooms and waterfall. We picked our room specifically for the private, two-steps-down entrance into the pool with a perfect view of the waterfall.

After lunch, we floated around the pool in our inner tubes and read our books. This was a great way to relax, get an even tan, and stay cool. Occasionally, we floated by the bar and grabbed a drink.

Our first full day, we had reservations at a very nice restaurant, The Cliff. The tables were widely dispersed on a cliff with magnificent views. When it was dark, lights below shone on a group of enormous stingrays swimming below. I wondered how they kept those stingrays there. *Are they imprisoned in a net or something? Do they feed them? I wonder what stingrays eat. Hmmm…*

Anyway, Mom and I ate at a secluded table, except for one other table on the cliff slightly above us. There sat a man eating alone who grinned and waved to us as we sat down. We smiled and waved back.

We had a lovely dinner supplemented with a nice bottle of chardonnay. When the man was finished with his dinner, he stopped by our table.

"Good evening, ladies," he greeted us.

"Hello! This is Vicki and I am Barbara," said my mom.

"I am Gabriel," the handsome, forty-something man introduced himself.

"Nice to meet you, Gabriel," I said smiling, shaking his hand, holding back the drool.

"Are you alone, Gabriel? Why don't you join us for a drink?" my shy mom asked the hunk.

"Only if you allow me to buy." *YES!*

So Gabriel proceeded to buy a bottle of champagne. A man after my own heart. Gabriel was in town on business. He was from Belgium and owned a waste management company. I was not sure what business someone in waste management would have in Barbados, but I didn't care. I liked Gabriel. So did Mom, "Gabriel, it looks like they are closing soon. Why don't you come back to our hotel for a drink?" *So smooth, Mom.*

"Great idea. The Colony Club is right next to my hotel. I would love to join you two lovely ladies."

The three of us took a cab back to the Colony Club and joined Laverne and Shirfeelia for a drink. After we ordered, Mom strategically yawned and said she was going to take hers back to the room. I had to chuckle. She was orchestrating this whole thing with Gabriel and me. Once alone, we took our drinks for a walk for some privacy. We sat talking by the water gently washing up on the shore with the moon brightly shining down. It was all very romantic, but I started getting nervous, even with the amount of liquid courage in my system. I was scared he was going to kiss me or notice my port or my wig or all of the above.

"Vicki, will you spend the day with me tomorrow? Why don't we have lunch? I will meet you at 11:00 a.m. over here, and we can walk down the beach to my place."

"Oh, that sounds perfect! I will see you right here at 11:00." It was then that he looked dreamily at me in the eyes. I knew it was coming. He kissed me. Softly at first, and then more passionately. Believe me. I kissed Gabriel right back and forgot about my cancer, my port, and my wig. *Isn't it always when you let your guard down that it happens?* Yes. He ran his hand through my wig and immediately discovered the truth. "Oh," was all he could say.

Embarrassed, I adjusted my wig and giggled nervously. "I guess I should have told you about my cancer. I have Hodgkin's lymphoma and am taking chemo. This is my wig and this is my port." I touched my wig and my port.

"Oh, Vicki. It surprised me, that's all. I am so sorry you have cancer. You look amazing, and I would never guess it."

"If you don't want to see me tomorrow, that's okay. I would understand."

"Don't be silly. What difference does it make? Unless it is too much for you. We could have lunch at your place."

"No! I would love to see your hotel. I will see you here at eleven, if you are still up for it?"

"Of course. Until then." He gave me a big smooch and walked off.

I received an inquisition from my supposedly tired mom when I returned to the room. She had to know everything. Okay. She deserved it for teeing the evening up perfectly.

As I fell asleep, I thought about Gabriel with a smile on my face. He felt wonderful in my arms. I had not kissed a man since I got sick.

It felt good, even with the wig screw-up. I was looking forward to the next day and thinking about what I was going to wear. I had a lingering thought in the back of my mind. *What if he doesn't show up?* It would be easy for him to blow me off. I decided to keep that thought in the back of my mind and think positively. I had a date with a dreamy Belgian tomorrow. *Could Gabriel be the man from far, far away?*

November 20, 2000

Mom and I woke up by the sunshine again. We looked out and saw Andrew cleaning the pool. He smiled and waved. We waved back. He motioned to us and the beach, signaling that he had saved our chairs. We thanked him and ate breakfast on our private patio. We gave Andrew a plate of food for breakfast too. He didn't want to be seen eating it, so we kind of slipped it to him. It seemed like he enjoyed it.

I tried to look extra good for my date. I tried on several bathing suits and cover-ups for my mom, kind of like a fashion show. I was convinced I had the best combo of suit, cover-up, and hat, and strolled out to our lounge chairs with an extra skip in my step.

As 11:00 a.m. rolled around, I had lost some confidence and the extra skip in my step as I convinced myself he wasn't coming. I was 50/50 on whether he would show. He was a nice guy, but who wants to deal with a bald, sick woman on vacation, if you don't have to?

He showed up at 11:05! Casually late. Nice.

"Good morning, Vicki! How are you this morning?" Gabriel gave me a hug and a kiss with a big beautiful smile.

"Good morning, Gabriel!" And we were off to walk down the beach to his hotel. We chatted as we walked down the beach. He grabbed my hand after a while. It was nice. I was actually happy I got the cancer thing out of the way. I tried to not talk about it, but it was hard because my cancer had been all consuming for the past six months. Even talking about work ended up talking about going on leave and chemo brain. I tried as hard as I could to focus on him in the conversation, diverting back to him when needed.

Gabriel was not actually at the hotel next door. He was staying in a villa. The villa was on a hill, overlooking the Caribbean. It was positively dreamy. We stood on his balcony and kissed. It was so romantic. Gabriel was a sweet kisser—nice and gentle.

Eventually, we ate lunch poolside. I was having a lovely time, but ever since the wig situation, it wasn't quite right. It's hard to explain.

After lunch, we hung out by the pool. We splashed, flirted, and kissed in the pool. Gabriel and I had fun, but again, it wasn't quite right.

Gabriel walked me home in the afternoon. The tide had risen. It was a difficult walk back through the water. I was glad I had him to help me as the waves crashed up on the rocks next to what previously was the beach. As we said goodbye, he gave me a sweet kiss and told me he would call me. We didn't make any specific plans but talked about going for a boat ride. He said he was going to investigate it, and let me know.

Again, I was 50/50 on whether he would call me. Typically, I would be more confident, but realistically, I didn't see where this was going. *Does he feel like it isn't quite right, also?*

I went back to the room and took a nap before dinner. I was exhausted. After about two hours, Mom woke me up and gave me the inquisition. We both decided not to think about whether he was going to call or not. Easier said than done.

Mom and I dined at The Tides in the nearby Holetown. Dinner was delicious. I was so happy to not have nausea. Food didn't quite taste the same, but it still tasted good. Everything had a slight metallic taste, even the chardonnay.

Mom and I went to the swim-up bar after dinner for a closer. We were excited to get off of the chardonnay train and have a Sambuca. Something different. Laverne gave us the clear alcohol in appropriate glasses.

"Do you have coffee beans?" I asked.

"What do you want coffee beans for?" Laverne responded.

"You are supposed to put three coffee beans in Sambuca for good luck," I said.

"Sorry, Vicki. We don't have any coffee beans."

Jokingly, I replied, "You are going to give me bad luck, Laverne."

My mom wouldn't even have the drink without coffee beans. "I will stick to chardonnay then."

"Okay. I will have your Sambuca." And I poured hers into mine to make one big Sambuca. More for me!

Back in the room, I checked for messages. None. Bummer.

November 21, 2000

The next morning, we woke up to rain. Pouring rain. That was the first sign of bad luck. It usually doesn't rain in Barbados—at least not like that. We decided to take a tour to Harrison's Cave, where there are stalactites and stalagmites. After my process and no call from Gabriel, we grabbed a cab to go to the cave.

We had barely gotten started down the long tree-lined driveway of the Colony Club when I fixed a bunched up sock in my shoe. Little did I know that my sock was not bunched up in my shoe. There was a three-inch cockroach in my shoe that was highly disturbed by my foot seeking shelter in its home.

"AHHHHH!!! Cockroach!" I screamed at the top of my lungs, with my mom quickly joining in upon seeing the invader.

The cockroach scurried all over the cab. The cab driver slammed on the breaks and joined us yelling. In unison, we all threw the doors open and jumped out of the cab. That gave the invader an opportunity to escape, as well.

By this time, bellmen came running down the driveway to save us from the attack. "Barbara, Vicki, are you all right?" they inquired, as they caught up with us.

"A six-inch cockroach was in Vicki's shoe!" Mom replied. The cockroach was huge, but not six inches. Mom tended to exaggerate.

The driver and the bellmen were both laughing. I was trying to recover from the scare.

"We are fine. Sorry to worry you," I said.

The excitement was all over, and we continued our journey to Harrison's Cave. It was pretty cool. I would recommend it for a rainy day, sans the cockroach.

We entered the cave in pouring rain. We exited the cave with a clear blue sky. "Our luck is changing!" I declared.

On the way back to the room, we saw a group of monkeys playing in the trees. They were adorable. It looked like they were a family of five ranging between one and three feet tall. I kept trying to get a picture of them with my camera, but they weren't coming out of the trees. Mom gave up. "I'm outta here. I am going to put on my suit."

"Okay. I'll give it five more minutes." I was determined to get a good picture.

After Mom left, they came out of the trees and were playing in front of me. I took a few pictures of them playing. While I focused on getting a good picture, one of them disappeared. The next thing I knew, *THUMP*. The wayward monkey jumped on my back and scared the shit out of me. "Aaahhhhhh!" I scared the shit out of it. The monkey jumped off of me and onto the railing next to me. *CLICK*. I took an amazing close-up picture of my attacker. *Success!*

By this time, not bellmen, but maids came running out to save me from my attacker. "Are you okay?" they asked me.

"Yes. I am fine. That monkey jumped on my back!" I explained. They acted like it was no big deal and went back to work.

Wow! The coffee bean thing is real! Three beans: rain, cockroach invasion, monkey attack. I went back to our room to change for the day.

I told Mom about the monkey attack and told her I had proof on my camera. She agreed with me about the bad luck.

Later, we floated around in the pool in our inner tubes while reading our books. We floated over to the bar and asked Laverne for a drink.

I couldn't help myself. "Laverne, remember how I told you it was bad luck to have Sambuca without three coffee beans? Well, I have been having bad luck all day." I proceeded to tell her all about the rain, the cockroach, and the monkey. She looked completely wide-eyed and spooked.

"Vicki, I didn't mean to give you bad luck! I am so sorry! What can I do to help?"

I was just joking around. I didn't mean to make her feel bad. She was very sorry.

"Oh, Laverne. I was just joking around. Don't worry about it. I'm fine, and you did nothing to me. It's okay."

My mom straightened me out later, "You know you really upset Laverne. They believe in all that voodoo crap down here. She thinks she cursed you or something."

Mom liked to stereotype.

November 22, 2000

Mom would do just about anything to make me happy, and she proved it over and over again. Today, she proved it once again with our excursion on the Jolly Roger.

A cab picked us up at the Colony Club to take us to Bridgetown. There we caught the ginormous, party, pirate ship for our three-hour cruise. As we boarded the ship, we were served rum punches via a keg. Mom just kept repeating herself, "I can't believe you are making me do this."

The Jolly Roger set sail. About a half an hour into the trip, we dropped anchor in a calm cove with clear, light blue water. While in the cove, the pirates made me walk the plank. They tried to take off my baseball cap, but I wasn't about to let that happen. I had no idea how high the plank actually was—like a couple stories high. Yikes!

My hat flew off as I plummeted into the water. I scrambled in the water to find it. Luckily, I found it floating nearby and snatched it up. It was really quite exhilarating. I swam to the back of the ship to find my mom.

Mom was on the deck getting some sun when I approached. "Mom, you have to walk the plank! It was so fun!"

"Oh, no you don't! I am not walking the plank! Leave me alone!"

"Aw, come on. You'll love it."

Just then, two pirates came to get Mom. "I am not doing this," she told them.

"Arrrrrrr. You have been very naughty, miss. Time to walk the plank! Arrrrr."

"How about swinging on the rope instead?" I asked. The rope swing wasn't so high up. *She actually went for it. Who knew?*

"Oh, no! Not the rope swing!" she cried to the pirates, playing along. And there you have it, Mom jumping off the pirate ship on a rope swing. I have the pictures to prove it! I couldn't wait to show her country club friends!

The Jolly Roger set sail again and took us to a coral reef. Passengers could snorkel or jet ski. After a quick inspection of the hygiene involved with mass quantities of people sharing snorkels and masks, we promptly picked the jet ski. Mom wanted me to drive, which I was happy to do.

We were pretty far from land. The huge, soft rolling waves allowed us to catch some air here and there. It felt so free. Exhilarating once again. I didn't have a care in the world, until my passenger started screaming in my ear, "Noooooo!"

I quickly stopped to check on her, "Are you all right?"

"Yes! This is great! Keep going!"

I sped up again, flying over the waves, as fast as the machine would go. "Nooooooo!" I heard from the peanut gallery in the back. Again, I stopped.

"What's going on?" I asked.

"Nothing. I am having a great time."

"Why do you keep saying 'no'?"

"I don't know."

"Well, stop it." And I sped off again to a peaceful silence, bouncing over the soft waves.

The Jolly Roger set sail again to return to Bridgetown. The passengers were pretty lit up as they danced the Macarena on the deck of the ship in their bikinis and thongs. It was fantastic people watching. The rum punch was long gone, and body shots were being served to the raunchy crowd. Mom decided two things: (1) She was the oldest one there, and (2) We were the only ones there without tats and body piercings.

All in all, even Mom would have to admit it was a fun day, minus the crowded, sweaty, dirty, loud, drunk, half-naked, tatted, pierced part.

It was dark by the time we got back to the Colony Club. I was beat. I was asleep before room service came with dinner. I never heard the door, Mom watching the TV, or Mom getting ready for bed.

November 23, 2000

The light creeped in and woke me up. I thought about yesterday and silently giggled. Then, I thought about Gabriel not calling me. It's too bad, but understandable. I shouldn't expect to meet my perfect man six months into chemo in Barbados. On the bright side, I had a very good time with Gabriel, while it lasted.

After the crazy day yesterday, we had a pretty chill day by the pool. Since Mom did the rope swing and the Jolly Roger for me, she got to make all the decisions for the day. It was Thanksgiving. What do you do on Thanksgiving in Barbados? You make reservations at an authentic Caribbean restaurant, Ragamuffins, for dinner and a show. Ragamuffins was down a dirt road, next to a local joint with people dancing in the street in the heart of Holetown. It was only 6:00 p.m., and the Barbadians were already dancing in the streets!

Ragamuffins was a small, casual restaurant with a bar, four stools, and a Caribbean vibe. I had a delicious West Indian curry dish that tasted like metal—go figure. I picked at my food while I checked out the small crowd of tourists waiting for the show. I couldn't figure out where the show was supposed to be. The place was so small. There was no room.

The drag show didn't need room for the entertainers to dance through the tables singing songs from Cher, Shania, Tina, and Barbra. Of course, Mom was an easy target for the interactive queens. She couldn't help but tell them how beautiful they were. They loved her.

After the show, we fought through the crowd dancing in the street to find a cab back to the hotel for a closer. No Sambuca this time. We had a glass of chardonnay with Laverne and Shirfeelia. Halfway through the glass of wine, the phone rang at the pool bar. Shirfeelia called out, "Barbara, telephone!" She passed the phone over to Mom. Mom was in shock.

"Who would be calling me?" She put the phone to her ear. "Hello?"

"Happy Thanksgiving, Mom!" Kristen had called to wish us a Happy Thanksgiving. When we didn't answer in the room, the front desk told Kristen we were out at the pool bar.

"How does the front desk know where you are?"

"I guess we are regulars at the pool bar," Mom guessed. It was three hours earlier in California.

Never a dull moment!

November 24, 2000

On our last full day, we wanted to make sure we took advantage of as much as possible at the Colony Club. Andrew saved our chairs for the morning on the beach. I swam out to the raft for a while. We snorkeled around the coral reef in front of our hotel. Mom walked down the beach. I couldn't walk very far, so I floated on a raft in the calm water.

A calypso band was playing by the pool for lunch. Mom and I got our Barbados punches and floated around the pool, listening to music, and reading our books. I wish I could have captured that moment in time and returned to it whenever I wanted. I forgot all about cancer and chemo.

We closed out our activities with a boat ride to see the sea turtles and sharks. I jumped in the water and swam with the turtles. Apparently, it was illegal to touch them, so I tried not to, but did by accident. There were several different kinds of turtles, ranging in size and color. Then, I swam with the sharks. Well, not really with them. They were in a large netted area that I swam around, checking them out. I didn't want to go any closer. Mom watched from the boat.

Afterward, we swam in our pool by the waterfall. That night we chilled out with Laverne and Shirfeelia before packing and hitting the hay early. *What an amazing busy week we had!*

November 25, 2000

I got up early on our last day. I met Andrew down by the beach as he was setting up the chairs. I read my book there until it was time to leave. It was time to go home to reality, cancer, and chemo. I had put it out of my mind, but it was back. Hopefully, I was done and could put cancer in the history books.

November 30, 2000

This was the big day I had been waiting for! *Is it gone?* I didn't think I could take any more chemo. Certainly not two more months of this hell. I had to be done.

Don't get me wrong; Mom's quest to entertain Vicki during this hell had been wonderful, but I felt like crap for most of it. I look at the pictures from our amazing trips, and I have a big smile on my face. That couldn't have been me. I don't look miserable in the pictures. That smile was masking my misery.

What I didn't share earlier was that I was puking all through Barbados. I puked on the plane. I puked at customs. I puked at The Cliff. I puked overboard on the Jolly Roger. I puked in the street outside Ragamuffins. I chose to not let my nausea ruin a good time. I chose not to think about it. I chose to have a glass half full. I chose to believe my cancer was gone, and I chose to be done with chemo.

Back to my big day. I did the full morning process, including my wake and bake. Mom took me to my appointment with Dr. Kim to receive the news on my all-important CT scan. If needed, I was going to stay and have chemo. If not, I was going to leave a very happy person. I was so nervous. I think Mom was too, because she was unusually quiet, which made me more nervous.

Dr. Kim started out with an examination, which made me wait a little longer. *Is she doing it on purpose? She has to know how anxious I am.* In fact, I told her. "I am anxious for my CT scan results. Is my cancer gone?" Now, *that* was direct. She kept examining me.

When the examination was finished, she was direct. "Your smaller tumor is gone, and your larger tumor has shrunk to a minimal size. All we see is scar tissue around your heart, but with it being minimal to nonexistent, I recommend four more treatments, starting today."

Ugh! This is a good news/bad news situation. I should be really happy, but instead, I just wanted to puke. I had a list of questions prepared for the appointment, but I didn't want to look at them. I quickly went from feeling half full to feeling half empty in a matter of seconds.

"I will do whatever you recommend, but are you sure? I really don't want any more chemo."

"Yes. I understand you don't want anymore, but it is better to be sure it is gone. You have three more after today. Can you do it?"

"Let's go for it!" And with that, Daniela shoved the IV in the port. She was all ready to go when we got there.

Mom had never been to a chemo before, not counting the first one. She had been to a lot of appointments and procedures with me, but this was the first chemo. I gave her my usual spiel.

I did the chemo trifecta: sleep, cry, puke. Mom witnessed the full monty.

We went home. I smoked some weed and slept until dinner.

Chapter Twelve

December 2000: My Remission!

> "The longer I live, the more beautiful life becomes."
> — Frank Lloyd Wright

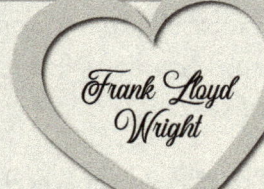

December 8, 2000

Since I told Dr. Kim I was having a shortness of breath, and she scheduled me for another pulmonary function test (PFT). The shortness of breath had increased since my last chemo. I had problems breathing, especially at night. I lay there in the dark, struggling to breathe, gasping for air. It kept me up at night. I kept thinking, *what if I stop breathing while I sleep? What if I don't wake up?* I didn't want to die because I fell asleep. I was not happy about this new symptom.

I went to the hospital for the PFT and another Neupogen shot. The Neupogen shot had become a part of my regimen.

The PFT was a complete failure and exposed my breathing problem. I guess it was proof to Dr. Kim that I actually had a problem and was not just complaining for the sake of complaining. I always had this feeling that I had to prove to Dr. Kim that there was actually something wrong with me and not just making shit up. *It is ridiculous. I have cancer for God's sake!*

December 14, 2000

I slept in and had a wake-and-bake session to kick off the morning. Mom had changed my baking location to the main-level powder room instead of the lower-level laundry room. Apparently, she no longer feared having her house smell like skunk. I had a late-morning chemo scheduled, so I took my sweet time with my process.

Heather picked me up for chemo. My levels were good, and the process started. Daniela informed me that I would not have any Bleomycin today due to my lung issue. I guess Bleomycin was the culprit that gave me the breathing problems. I was also told that if my breathing got worse, I might have to go on a respirator. *Yikes!*

I felt so weak and tired when I talked to Dr. Kim. My writing in my journal was so sloppy you could barely read my notes. She wanted me to increase the Prednisone for my lung issue. I had just weaned down on it, and now I had to take more. We also discussed my new problem—anal abscess.

This disease gets better all of the time. Apparently, I developed an infection in my butt. Dr. Kim referred me to a proctologist. I had to schedule an appointment to have it lanced. As if I didn't have enough problems. *How humiliating!*

Besides the lung and butt discussions and absence of Bleomycin, chemo was typical: sleep, puke, cry. *My hat trick.*

December 20, 2000

Kristen, Bryan, and Kirby came to town for Christmas. We always have a very festive time at Christmas, much more festive than in Orange County, so they came to the cold. The first festive thing to do was to take me to have my abscess lanced. Kristen volunteered and had the pleasure of escorting me to the hospital for the lancing. It was considered a surgical procedure.

Kristen sat in the waiting room while I was prepped for surgery. I had a fun IV going when a fellow club member walked by to say hi. "Fitz" was an orthopedic surgeon. "Good morning, Vicki. What brings you in today?" Fitz asked while reading my chart. "Oh, I see."

Luckily, the fun IV cocktail kicked in, so I chuckled. "Hi, Fitz."

"Good luck today." He grinned.

That's just what I needed. I hope he remembered the Hippocratic Oath. I had enough people talking about my cancer. I didn't need people talking about my butt.

The lancing went fine, and Kristen brought me home for a nap. It was cold and snowing—typical December day in Chicago. We were supposed to go to a Bulls game that night, and I wasn't so sure we were still going if it was five degrees and a negative wind-chill. I set my alarm anyway.

"So what does the team think about the game tonight?" I said as I headed to the ganja room.

"I want to go!" Kirby chimed in. "I want to see Michael Jordan!"

"Michael's not playing anymore," Kristen informed her. "Vicki, are you up to it? We could go without you. Or I could stay home with you. I'm not so sure I want to go out in this weather."

"Ask me again in a minute," I yelled from the bathroom, while taking a drag. Two puffs did the trick. I left the bathroom, smelling like a skunk.

"Aunt Vicki farted!" Kirby cried out.

"Sorry, guys. I smelled up the bathroom. I think I am good to go."

Bryan added, as he headed into the ganja room, "I don't mind the smell."

"Yuck," answered Kirby.

So we piled into Mom's car and went downtown to the United Center. Even with the handicap parking, we had a horrendous walk to get to the stadium in the freezing cold. The snow was blowing sideways, like a blizzard. I gripped Bryan's arm as hard as I could while he dragged me down the sidewalk to the gate. I regretted not being on the couch with a fire. *Why did I say yes to this madness? Why did I put myself through this misery?*

Once we were in the stadium, my attitude changed. The vibe in the stadium put us all in a good mood, even Mom. My mom and I splurged on good Bulls tickets a few times a year, starting in the

Jordan era. The team stunk this year, but the entertainment value was still there. Luckily, once in the stadium, I didn't have very far to walk.

The Bulls lost to the Pacers, but at least it was competitive. We usually leave after the game ends, but we ended up leaving a little early to beat traffic and get me home. The snow turned off some of the crowd, so it definitely wasn't a full stadium. I was home in bed in thirty minutes.

December 24, 2000

I slept in and was relieved my roommate did the same. Kirby was a fun roommate. She babbled up a storm while getting ready for bed. Luckily, once in bed, she slept like a log. I lay there gasping for air, wondering if I was going to make it through the night, while she slept peacefully. I was exhausted from all of the running around, so I didn't lie there too long before I fell asleep. When we woke up, I had to reassure an anxious Kirby that it wasn't Christmas yet. She always put a smile on my face. It's wonderful to wake up to that pure energy.

We went downstairs to a bustling kitchen full of breakfast smells. Kristen and Bryan were making eggs and bacon, which sent me flying into the bathroom to dry heave. I returned after my morning smoke. I passed on the eggs, preferring my usual Raisin Bran. Then I headed over to the couch with a pit stop to my smoke station. Even though we had a lot of activities scheduled, I retained a number of my process steps and habits. I had a bath on the agenda later in the day after Christmas movies.

Having my family in for Christmas certainly raised my spirits, but it was exhausting. I had become "Vegetable Vicki" who spent the day horizontal, only getting vertical to move from the bed to the bathroom to the couch or to the bathtub. Those were my days. When they came into town, that rocked my mojo, but I went with it. I tried hard and put a smile on my face. Fake it until you make it!

Cancer has very few upsides to it. One of those upsides happened to be skipping church on Christmas Eve. The other girls went to 3:00 p.m. mass, while Bryan and I stayed home. Not that I disliked church, but we typically ended up leaving the house an hour early to sit in the pew for fifty minutes waiting for mass to start. I was happy to avoid that. Bryan wasn't Catholic, so he also got a pass.

After church, the gang picked Bryan and me up to go to our cousin's house for our family Christmas party. This tradition started with my dad's family over forty years ago. The crew consisted of about twenty-five adults and twenty-five kids, most of which were on the raft trip in Idaho. Santa always stopped by to say hi and leave presents for the kids on his route around the world. Bryan had his stint as Santa, because most of the kids didn't recognize him, coming from Orange County. He was getting pretty good at it.

My cousin Pat had the party at his house, which was decked out for Christmas with a two-story Christmas tree. Everything was first class from the Dom Perignon to the beef tenderloin.

After we were at the party for about an hour, Bryan went upstairs to suit up and study the kids' names. Suddenly, there was a commotion coming from the front of the house and everyone started screaming for Santa like he was a rock star. Santa walked in with a full sack of gifts, courtesy of Barbara. Mom loved buying the gifts for the kids. She worked really hard on getting the right thing for the right age.

The kids were hanging on to Santa. He needed bodyguards to protect him and his false beard. Kristen stepped in and took over as bodyguard, shooing the kids away. One by one, Santa called the kids up to sit on his lap and give them a present. He got a few screamers, but that was par for the course. After the kids, the ladies got their chance to sit on Santa's lap. Santa always got fresh with a particular lady.

The party doesn't last very long due to cranky kids and busy schedules. We had to get home, put some milk and cookies out for Santa, and go to bed. Kirby and I headed upstairs, while the rest of the team finished wrapping their presents. Kirby was all wound up and not ready for bed. I stopped listening as she wondered out loud about potential presents. Actually, the babble helped me to forget about my breathing.

December 25, 2000

Around 8:00 a.m., I felt a nudge followed by a giggle. It was Kirby nudging me awake. "Is it time yet?"

"Just about," I replied, as I slowly got up. I loved Christmas.

We huddled at the top of the stairs until we got the high sign to come down. The stockings over the fireplace were bulging with little presents. The wee one yelled, "Santa came!" *Was there any doubt?*

After we opened the stocking presents, we had some coffee cake for breakfast and a mimosa to wash it down. Mom ordered me to the smelly bathroom before we continued down to the lower level to open presents under the tree. We were done by 9:30 a.m., giving us the whole day to play with new toys, try on new clothes, watch Christmas movies, or, in my case, take a bath and a nap.

My mom's aunt Willa always gave us wacky presents ever since we were kids. She still sent us nutty stuff. This year, Kirby got a set of fake mustaches. "What are these for?" she asked her mom.

"Good question, Kirby. Maybe she wanted us to wear them for Christmas dinner?" Kristen replied. *I'm not sure what crazy Aunt Willa was thinking either.*

"Oh yeah. That makes sense." Kirby nodded. *Huh? It makes sense?* She took out the mustaches and handed each of us one to put on. We wore them for the rest of the night, posing and taking pictures.

We had so much fun with these mustaches, trying to eat and drink with them, etc. *Maybe there is a point to Kirby's gift?*

Kirby and I went to bed after watching *It's a Wonderful Life*. I fell asleep during the movie, but I know the ending. Her babbling about her gifts put me to sleep again, avoiding the nasty breathing. I wished Kirby could be my roommate all of the time.

I woke myself up in the middle of the night gasping for air. I was okay. Then, I started remembering my dream. In the dream, I watched my family live without me, like I died, or never existed. Damn movie!

Mom was remarried and had my sister in town for Christmas to stay with them in a huge house. Bryan and Kirby were nowhere to be seen. Mom's new husband was REALLY old and cranky. She was running around serving his every last whim. Kristen had a Southern accent and came in from Texas. Life was really different without me. I tried to make sense of it all, but it didn't make sense. I guess one might have said I was somehow responsible for Kristen and Bryan getting married and for my mom not getting married again. Unfortunately, this notion, along with my infiltrated lungs, kept me from getting a good sleep.

December 28, 2000

The California crew was back in the OC, and I went to my fifteenth chemo. I couldn't believe I was almost to the finish line! One more to go after today!

Julie took me to chemo. While I was busy or sleeping, she walked around the hospital and caught up with some of her friends from work. I was pretty much Vegetable Vicki. I completed my trifecta, and Dr. Kim walked in.

"Good morning, Vicki. How are you doing today?"

"Okay. Tired. Nauseous."

"Well, you are almost across the finish line. One more to go. Think of it this way for the New Year: you are in remission. The chemo in January is just precautionary. Be happy."

Imagine her telling me to be happy! *Hmmm. Not sure what to do with that one.*

"I will be happy to get this over with," I replied, forcing a smile. I guess that wasn't very nice. I added, "So, I really am in remission?"

"Yes, Vicki. You are in remission."

I gave her a big Vicki grin. "Thank you. Happy New Year!"

December 31, 2000

New Year's Eve started out with my usual morning wake-and-bake process. Everything Mom and I did today was late, so we could stay up until midnight. After smoking my weed, I wrote a detailed entry in my journal regarding the conclusion of my millennium.

As with every year, I reviewed how I finished on all of my goals for the year and set new goals for the upcoming year. It gave me a special time to reflect on the year's ups and downs, while setting myself up for a successful new year.

2000 Goals:

1) **Men:** The year began strong on the dating scene, but ended up nowhere pretty quickly. Goal—fail. Never mind. It's too hard to meet someone in the middle of a cancer battle. I gave myself a pass. **Goal—meets expectations.** I will transfer it to my 2001 goals.
2) **Career:** Success in the first quarter but couldn't hang on due to circumstances beyond my control. Goal—fail. Scratch that. I moved on with my career. **Goal—meets expectations.** I will transfer it to my 2001 goals.
3) **Health:** What unexpectedly became my biggest focus of the year, I failed tremendously and then rebounded quite nicely for the win. My goal was to lose ten pounds, and I lost seventeen. I gave myself major health bonus points for overcoming the cancer I didn't know I had. I was in remission! Even though I had one more chemo left, I was in remission! **Goal—exceeds expectations.** I kicked ass! 2001 goal: solve numb, throbbing, weak extremity issues.

I had a late-afternoon bath with Harry Potter. Coincidentally, I was reading the last book as I finished my millennium journey. Harry had been through a lot, as I read page after page in the tub. And so have I. I thought about being in remission but having one more chemo to go. *Why should I do it? Haven't I had enough? Is there a point? Is there some hard rule that you had to have six or eight months exactly? Is it a gold standard that doctors can't vary the protocol at all?* Trying to get the right frame of mind, I tried to justify it. I searched for an analogy. Maybe it was like shooting your enemy (cancer), and you knew it was dead, but you took one more shot for the finality of it all. I went with it. Kill the asshole! And take *that* for good measure!

The evening was quite different this year—no hick bars, no screaming kids, no hanging out with couples, no Y2K threat. No corporation. Pretty tame. Mom and I had some champagne, like last year, but everything else was different. I was pretty sick from the chemo that I had a few days earlier, but the ganja took care of that.

After my extra-long bath with Harry, I took an extra-long nap. Mom cooked an amazing steak dinner. We discussed remission, my last chemo, and my analogy. Mom shared with me that she secretly started planning another Vicki Trip.

"As soon as Dr. Kim gives us the okay, let's jump in the car and drive down to Florida for the month. We can stop at a bunch of places and see some friends."

Wow! I was surprised, excited, thrilled, and touched. I was so suddenly slammed with emotion that my eyes started to tear up. "Really? I would love to do that! Where would we go?"

"I have been thinking about it for a while. Let's drive down Tampa or Orlando, then Naples to see the Thompsons, then Jupiter to see the cousins, then Ft. Lauderdale to see Millicent (my grandmother). We could jump over to Atlantis in the Bahamas for a few days and start making our way home."

"That sounds absolutely amazing! I'm in!"

Now that was exactly what I needed. I was a little scared of the future. I was thinking about the limbo after chemo. After being so highly focused on beating cancer, I hadn't thought much about what I was going to do next. This trip would be a nice way to relax, heal, and think about the future. I needed to get the poison out of me and gain strength. I was so incredibly weak. I would come back from Florida, cancer-free, poison-free, nausea-free, chemo brain-free, strong, and ready to take on life again.

We watched *The Godfather* on TV to take us to the finish line. I tried to get Mom to smoke weed with me after dinner. She took a hard pass.

"Come on, Mom. You used to smoke cigarettes every day. Don't you want to see what pot is like?"

"No, Vicki, I am not smoking your little thing."

"No one will know. I won't tell anyone."

"I don't succumb to peer pressure."

"Pretty please. Do it for me," I kept trying.

"I said, NO!"

Okay. I tried. I thought she would give in. So, I got high by myself and took an extra hit to celebrate the New Year. *I wonder how much longer I will keep up my new drug habit?*

When *The Godfather* was over, we watched the countdown at Navy Pier. I was in and out of sleep during the movie and bounced awake for the countdown. I was wide awake and ready to toast the end of the year. Put this one to bed. Mom and I reminisced about the year as we poured a glass of champagne. I was in remission, and we had something to celebrate. I could move on with my life and look at my millennium in the rearview mirror.

10, 9, 8, 7, 6, 5, 4, 3, 2, 1, HAPPY NEW YEAR!

My millennium was over.

Epilogue

> "Often, when you think you're at the end of something, you're at the beginning of something else."
> — *Fred Rogers*

My millennium was not the year I intended it to be, but life rarely ends up the way you intended. I was supposed to be married with two kids, a dog, and a picket fence by the time I was thirty-four.

Life is filled with ups and downs and is what you make of it. Cherish the ups, and plow through the downs until you find yourself in a good place again. I certainly had a lot of ups and downs in 2000. I like to focus more on the positive. In that case, my millennium was filled with wonderful moments that I will cherish forever.

What doesn't kill you makes you stronger? I suppose I am stronger for my millennium. *How did my millennium change my life?* I am not thoroughly sure. I did not have an epiphany or anything. I think my biggest "come to Jesus moment" was in Alabama at the hotel basking in my misery. Bryan was the recipient of that phone call filled with self-pity.

I am sure everyone's experience with cancer is different. Everyone has some takeaways from their experience. My experience left me wanting to write a book for closure, as well as to help newly diagnosed patients by sharing my experience. I hope I helped you by writing this book. It helped me by writing it.

I learned a lot about dealing with cancer.

- Talking with someone with the same type of cancer and chemo protocol helped make me feel more comfortable with my journey.
- Bonding with others going through treatment at the same time helped lift my spirits and provide a sense of community.
- Writing in my journal helped me remember everything for doctor visits and understand patterns and feelings.
- Experiencing people avoiding me like a leper helped me understand that it is important to talk to others experiencing a health crisis.
- Allowing my friends to help me included them in my journey and improved my moods.
- Smoking pot really helped me with nausea.
- Managing your health is your responsibility. If something doesn't feel right, be diligent in figuring out what is going on.
- Being mindful, grateful, and positive can help your spirits.
- Finding alternative solutions can help.
- Doing fun things that you find joy in can make your journey more pleasurable.

Writing *My Millennium* was cathartic for me. It helped with my mom's recent passing. Our relationship was unique, but a lot of women can identify with my "mommy" issues and can relate. I treasure the time we spent together during my millennium. She succeeded in making my millennium more pleasant with lots of terrific times. In fact, I enjoyed a lot of it. Writing the book reminded me of all of the ways my mom loved and supported me, even if she had a hard time showing it on a daily basis. My cancer diagnosis really rocked her world.

During Mom's final months, I am glad that I could be there for her when she needed me, as she was there for me through my health crisis. We went to Barbados a few more times and hung out with Laverne and Shirfeelia. I tried to make her comfortable near the end and respect her wishes. Mom loved and appreciated me and my support, which took me a long time to realize. She would be very proud of me finishing my book, as my dad would be.

It is now 2024, and I would like to give you an update on my three millennium goals.

Health: I am pleased to announce that, in 2024, I am still in remission—almost twenty-five years later! I couldn't be happier about it! What a relief! Although, I never solved my extremity issue. Hopefully, someone will someday. While the issue is much better, I still experience it from time to time. I did see Dr. Posner, the great doctor, at Sloan Kettering, and participated in a Rockefeller University study on paraneoplastic syndromes. The diagnosis was neither confirmed nor denied. My lungs cleared up in early 2001. I stopped smoking pot on the Florida trip with my mom. My health certainly has been up and down over the years, but the forecast is sunny! AND, I always want to lose those ten pounds.

Men: I failed again in 2001, but I met my handsome, warmhearted millennium man at my club in 2004 and have been married sixteen years. It took me a while to find Greg, but I am so happy to find the man I love so deeply. He is my best friend, supporter, and life partner. While we travel a lot, we have never lived far, far away, as the fortune-teller suggested. In fact, we live in the same town that I grew up in. I have two lovely stepdaughters in the area. Greg is an extravert accountant with a love of sports, golf, and fun. No picket fence with two kids and a dog, but a wonderful life nevertheless. I can't imagine life without him. Conventional and unconventional at the same time. We try to live life to the fullest. Live! Love! Laugh!

Career: I made some money from the sale of the start-up, but it did not make me the millionaire Kirby was hoping for. I toyed with the idea of working for the Salt Lake Olympics as the director of communications, until I found out I wasn't going to be skiing every day and was expected to be working twelve-hour days. Eventually, I went back to the corporation and became the director I wanted to be. I never worked as hard as I did during my pre-cancer years, with one exception: a project that had me working twenty-hour days for over a month. Believe me; it's not worth it. I retired from the corporation after thirty years. I even consulted for them for a few years, in retirement.

My supportive friends and cousins still remain tight in my life. Now their kids are getting married and having kids of their own. My friend with Hodgkin's, Jeff, and I stayed in touch for a few years, both staying in remission. While I never set out to run marathons, Jeff continued to do so. I really admire his strength. My mom's friends, Nancy and Diane, eventually both passed away from cancer. I hope they knew how much they inspired me through my journey.

I am not sure what happened to Alan, Larry, Christian, Bill, Craig, and Gabriel, my millennium men. I do know that Craig, the pianist, went to Afghanistan and came home a hero to his wife and kids.

Kristen and Bryan eventually moved to Dallas a few years ago. They are looking forward to retiring someday soon. They are enjoying life, golfing year round and traveling whenever they can. Kirby graduated from Southern Methodist University with an engineering degree and is a consultant at Ernst & Young in Chicago. We still go on our family ski trips.

Greg and I retired early and are living in Glenview. I love him so much. We have a lot of the same interests and love sharing our lives together. We spend a lot of time with our philanthropies. We play golf at our club where I often end up in the dreaded eighth-hole sand trap. I still have the angel Heather gave me on my nightstand looking over me. I still go to Sunday Funday with Cynthia and Margie's families. Some things never change.

Y2K issues were supposed to make the millennium year a complete disaster. All hell was supposed to break loose when computers failed around the world. We were all prepared for the worst to happen. Instead, it was no big deal. But "my millennium" was a big deal to me. All of the Y2K preparations did not help me prepare for my millennium personal crisis. My hope is that *My Millennium* helps you prepare for your own personal crisis.

With the physical and emotional roller-coaster rides, I will never forget my millennium. *How could I?* The incredible bond with Mom, the health crisis, the misery, the fun, the struggles, the highs, the lows, and the hilarious wacky times make my millennium unforgettable. My millennium set me up for the rest of my wonderful life.

Acknowledgments

Thank you to my friends and family who supported me through my cancer journey. Your support made my millennium the best that it could have been. Thank you for taking me to my treatments. Thank you for taking me to doctors' appointments. Thank you for taking me to procedures. Thank you for taking me to lunch and dinner. Thank you for your advice. Thank you for getting me out. Thank you for your companionship. Thank you for your hugs. Thank you for your cards. Thank you for your flowers. Thank you for your love!

Thank you to Cate, Colleen, Cynthia, Diane, Heather, Heather Mac, Hodie, Hugh, Jamie, Jeff, Julie, Karen, Kurt, Margie, Nancy, Pam, Robin, Sharon, and Sue. Thank you to those I forgot to mention.

Thank you to my doctors and nurses. Your support got me to remission. Thank you for your healing powers. Thank you Daniela, Dr. Kim, Dr. Liptay, Dr. Randall, Dr. Revis, and Dr. Zaacks.

Thank you to my millennium men. You guys are awesome—Alan, Bill, Christian, Craig, Gabriel, and Larry.

Thank you to the corporation and the start-up for your patience and support.

Thank you to Kristen, Bryan, and Kirby, whose love, support, and visits were incredibly helpful in my journey.

Thank you to Mom, my partner in this fight.

Thank you to Greg, my best friend, partner, husband, #1 fan, reviewer, and soul mate. Thank you for hanging with me through the dusting off and finishing of my book. Your encouragement and love mean the world to me.

Thank you to Greg, Jamie, Julie, Kate, Margie, and Susan, who helped me throughout the publishing process. AND, thanks to Sarah, my inspiration to finally finish *My Millennium*!

Printed in the USA
CPSIA information can be obtained
at www.ICGtesting.com
JSHW081120051124
72825JS00003B/3/J